SEX, SEX, *and More* SEX

ALSO BY SUE JOHANSON

*Sex Is Perfectly Natural,
but Not Naturally Perfect*

Talk Sex

[SUE JOHANSON]

SEX, SEX, *and*
More SEX

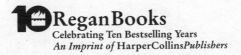
ReganBooks
Celebrating Ten Bestselling Years
An Imprint of HarperCollins*Publishers*

This book contains advice and information relating to health care. It is not intended to replace medical advice and should be used to supplement rather than replace regular care by your doctor. It is recommended that you seek your physician's advice before embarking on any medical program or treatment. All efforts have been made to assure the accuracy of the information contained in this book as of the date of publication. The publisher and the author disclaim liability for any medical outcomes that may occur as a result of applying the methods suggested in this book.

HarperCollins books may be purchased for educational, business, or sales promotional use. For information please write: Special Markets Department, HarperCollins Publishers Inc., 10 East 53rd Street, New York, NY 10022.

Designed by Kris Tobiassen

ISBN 0-06-056666-3

To all the people who
made my career "just happen"

Contents

Acknowledgments *xi*

Introduction *1*

A

Abortion *5*

Affairs *6*

After Sex *10*

Aging and Sex *11*

AIDS *19*

Anal Sex *26*

Anger *30*

Anorexia *33*

Aphrodisiacs *34*

B

Battering: Abused Men *39*

Battering: Abused Women *40*

Bisexuality *46*

Bladder Infection *49*

Bondage and Discipline *51*

Boredom *52*

Breaking Up *53*

Breasts, Female *60*

Breasts, Male *61*

C

Celibacy *62*

Circumcision, Female *64*

Circumcision, Male *67*

Cock Rings *70*

Condoms *71*

Contraception Advances *74*

Cysts, Ovarian *78*

D

Depression 81
Disability 84
Doctor/Therapist–Client
    Abuse 86

E

Ectopic Pregnancy 89
Endometriosis 91
Erotica and Pornography 95
Expectations 98

F

Faking Orgasm 101
Fantasy 104
Fetal Alcohol Syndrome 107
Fetish 108
Fibroids 110
Flirting 111
Forgiveness 114
Frequency 117
Fun Sex 121

G

G-Spot 123
Gender Selection 127
Guilt 129

H

Hairiness 133
Headache 134
Homosexuality 136
Hysterectomy 144

I

Impotence (Erectile
    Dysfunction) 148
Incest 150
Incontinence 153
Infertility 155
Internet
    Pornography 163
Internet Sex 164

J

Jealousy 165

K

Kegel Exercises 167

L

Low Sex Drive 170
Low Sperm Count 171

M

Masturbation 173
Meeting "Someone" 176
Menopause, Female 177
Menopause, Male
    (Andropause) 180
Middle Years, The 182
Miscarriage 184
Morning-after Pill 188

O

Office Relationships 190
Oral Sex 193

Orgasm 196
Osteoporosis 198

P

Pap Smear 201
Penis Size 204
Peyronnie's Disease
    206
Phone Sex 208
Piercing 210
Piles (Hemorrhoids) 211
Positions 212
Power/Control 214
Pregnancy 218
Premature Ejaculation 224
Premenstrual Syndrome
    225
Prolapsed Uterus 227
Prostate Tumors 228
Prostatic Stimulation 230
Prostitution 230

R

Relationships 232
Retarded (Delayed)
    Ejaculation 236

S

Self-Concept Self-Esteem
    239
Sex Addiction 242
Sexual Assault 245

Sexually Transmitted
    Diseases 249
    Chlamydia 249
    Gonorrhea 250
    Hepatitis B 252
    Herpes Simplex 253
    Venereal Warts 256
Sex Toys 257
    Ben Wah Balls 257
    Vibrators 258
Shy Man Syndrome 259
Smoking 262
Sterilization 264
Stretch Marks 267
Syphilis 268

T

Threesomes 270
Tipped Uterus 272
Touching 273
Trust 275

U

Unconsummated Sex 279
Uterine Ablation 282

V

Vaginal Farts 283
Virginity 284

Y

Yeast Infection 287

Acknowledgments

I've heard it said that "life is what happens to you when you plan something else." This book developed that way, and I would like to thank all the people who made it happen. My thanks to the people at Penguin Books for believing that Susie can and will do it, and for allowing me to do it my way. I am especially grateful to Cynthia Good, who recognized that I do not need outlines and deadlines. She just let me be, which was wonderful. And thanks as well to editors Nicole de Montbrun of Penguin Canada and Cassie Jones of Regan-Books USA.

My thanks to Dr. Stephen Holzapfel, who reviewed the book and filled in the gaps in information from the medical/counseling perspective; and to Margaret Jacobs, an Ottawa-based sex educator, counselor, and therapist, who reviewed the manuscript and added some valuable insights. Their expertise ensured accuracy and balanced a topic that is so often "out of whack."

Number one in my life is my family, who simply regard my career as the most natural happening. They are impressed but not awed by it, and they provide the absolute unconditional acceptance that we all need in our lives.

Finally, a special thanks to all the listeners and viewers who inspired me to write this book for those who are unable to obtain information that some consider explicit and controversial.

I hope you enjoy reading *Sex, Sex, and More Sex* as much as I have enjoyed writing it.

Introduction

If your sex life is important to you, and if you want to make it good and keep it that way, this book is for you.

It could be subtitled "Sex Simplified," because that is exactly what I want the book to do: to make it as easy as possible to get answers to the most commonly asked questions about sex—no hassle, no sweat, and no embarrassment. This is why I chose to alphabetize the book. Just "let your fingers do the walking"—it's as simple as using a phone book.

I learned very little about sex when I was a teen, and training to be a nurse in a Catholic hospital in Winnipeg did little to expand my knowledge base. But raising teens does not allow you the luxury of denial that they are sexual. When one of my children's classmates confided she had missed her period, the importance of extensive sex education and the availability of birth control became paramount to me. I set up and ran a teen clinic in the health room of a local high school, staffed by volunteer doctors and nurses. During my time there I came to a realization: while most people have a basic understanding of human sexuality—what I call "the plumbing of sex"—the "acts, facts, and feelings" are not something you learn about in Sex Ed 101.

The clinic was well received by teens. So, it was back to college to get the necessary skills to teach sex ed. As a sex educator, I encouraged my students to write out questions about sex, anonymously, and I would answer them at the end of every class. I kept these "Dear Sue" question cards, organized them into topics, alphabetized them, and wrote out the answers. These cards were the beginning of *Sex, Sex, and More Sex*.

Later, for twelve years I hosted a popular, syndicated two-hour phone-in radio show on a Canadian rock radio station every Sunday. In 1986 I hosted a weekly TV show. Between the two shows I receive piles of mail from wonderful men and women who want information and book lists.

Trying to keep up with the demand, over the years I wrote a series of handouts on a wide variety of topics, ranging from sexual abuse to yeast infections. Some handouts were in greater demand than others—oral-genital sex (blow job, going down on, giving head) was the most requested, followed by the Pill, the G-spot, and then anal sex.

Today, I do presentations at universities, and every student who attends is given a "Dear Sue" question card. I still make time to answer every question at the end of my talk and on my show, taking questions from callers across North America.

With all these questions in mind, I decided to incorporate the most popular topics into a book. In an effort to keep it simple, I use everyday language with no medical terminology unless it is explained, and I also use street language, or slanguage. For many topics, I mention a terrific book or two that covers a particular subject in more detail.

Recently there have been a plethora of books on "flavor of the day" topics such as orgasm and G-spot orgasm, anal sex, Viagra, low sex drive, menopause, and andropause. But there have been very few good books about communication and relationships, so some of the books I suggest as resources are oldies but goodies. You should be able to order them from a bookstore or Amazon.com, or you may find them at used bookstores or garage sales.

Because of the risk of AIDS and other sexually transmitted infections (STIs), I emphasize the importance of practicing Safer Sex. (The only safe sex is no sex or masturbation.) I frequently use the term "partner," which can mean anyone in any type of relationship. Many of the questions people have in same-sex relationships are similar to those in heterosexual ones. In cases where I feel therapy could be useful, I frequently suggest that you do some homework, such as keeping a journal, while you are looking for a counselor. You can buy an inexpensive, lined notebook, and start spilling your feelings out on paper. You do not have to worry about grammar, punctuation, spelling, or continuity. Nobody reads this but you. Writing in a journal helps many people to focus and clarify their feelings. Once you have these feelings down on paper, you stop reviewing them over and over again in your head. And when you go back and reread the writings, you will likely discover that you have gained the insight to deal with the realities of your life. It must be clear that this is *your* journal; nobody has the right to read it; it is private and confidential. Make it very clear that you will not be responsible for anyone's reactions if they read your journal.

Contrary to the "happily-ever-after" Hollywood movies, loving, caring, human sexual relationships do not just happen—they require work. The work involves good communication in a committed, trusting, honest manner. I hope you and your partner will each read this entire book, and then read it aloud together and discuss it as you go along. My best to you; may your partner be your best friend as well as your lover.

[a]

ABORTION

Dear Sue: *I am from a religious background, and I really believed that abortion was murder—that it was a crime and a sin. Then, in my second year of college, I got pregnant. Marriage was out of the question. I knew I could never give up a baby for adoption, so I chose abortion. For about two years I was consumed by guilt. Fortunately, the abortion clinic provided excellent postabortion counseling, and I finally got the help I needed. I graduated, have a good job, got married, and have two magnificent kids. Although I sometimes think about that pregnancy with sadness, I don't regret the decision I made, and I don't feel guilty. I was lucky. Please tell others to go for help.*

Sue says: What more can I say? Remorse over the abortion could have had a devastating effect on your life, but you had counseling. Usually, clinics offer counseling that helps women examine their value system and look at the messages they were given as children. Provided accurate information, these women are then able to make a decision about what is best for them at that stage of their life. In your case, such counseling helped you move beyond guilt and to appreciate your life as it is in the present.

Unfortunately, many women may experience postabortion guilt. For them, I strongly recommend short-term counseling to help them deal with their feelings. I am aware that abortion is a very controversial issue and must remain a personal choice. Nobody has the right to impose his or her morals on anyone else.

You might find the following book of some help: *The Gynecological Sourcebook* by M. Sara Rosenthal (New York: McGraw-Hill, 2003), 4th ed.

AFFAIRS

Dear Sue: *My wife had an affair with one of the men at her office. She says it's over now, but I just can't put it out of my mind. What does he have that I don't? I keep wondering if I am as good as he was, so I can't get an erection. How could she do that to me?*

Now I have to be honest and tell you that I had a little fling myself shortly after our son was born, but it meant nothing to me. She was upset for a while, but she got over it. What should I do?

Sue says: First, I would never tell you what you should do. I'll give you information and some insight into what might be happening, and you can examine your alternatives and decide how you want to deal with this problem.

Recent surveys indicate that there has been a dramatic increase in the number of women who instigate divorce action. There are several reasons for this.

- Women have expectations of what a loving relationship should add to life, and if their own marriage does not meet these expectations, they try to meet them by having an affair.
- Women's opportunities to meet other men have increased because they are in the workplace meeting "new and interesting" males.
- Women are more financially independent, so the prospect of being left with no financial support is not as scary.

Other possible reasons for women's extramarital affairs are:

- Romance—the magic has vanished from the marriage, the honeymoon is over, so they look for it elsewhere.
- An ego boost—to prove she is still attractive, that she can get a man.
- Revenge—to get even or to punish a partner for some indiscretion.
- The marriage is over anyway, so why not?
- A onetime mistake—she got carried away, it just happened.
- Curiosity—to try sex in new and different ways.
- Risk taking—to see what she can get away with, to push her luck.
- Rebellion—"I'll show you, you can't control me."
- Loneliness—feeling isolated.

Do any or all of these explanations apply to your partner and you? Have you noticed that she did not react as strongly to your outside affair as you did to hers? This is not uncommon—as much as we've accomplished in gender equality, society still has double standards when it comes to extramarital affairs. Many women still assume that "boys will be boys," that men are "victims" of "toxic testosterone." I believe many women still initially accept a husband's indiscretion as long as he doesn't repeat it. This does not mean that women forgive and forget, they don't—unless their husband appears totally repentant. Your wife may not have confided in you about the depth of her feeling when you cheated on her, and may be having an affair to get back at you.

Do you think it is more acceptable for men to have affairs than for women? Some women still buy into the idea that men are not genetically programmed to be monogamous. But in our society, most women expect that their partner will be faithful. For insight into your situation, do read *After the Affair: Healing the Pain and Rebuilding Trust When a Partner Has Been Unfaithful* by Janis Abrahms Spring, Ph.D., with Michael Spring (New York: Perennial, 1997). Abrams found that if a man initiates a divorce, he is likely to claim that it's because his wife has had an extramarital affair. However, if the wife sues for divorce, the cause is probably mental, physical, emotional, or sexual cruelty or abuse.

Here are more interesting observations about women involved in extramarital affairs.

- Women see and hear of other women having affairs, and there is the bandwagon effect—since everybody else is doing it, they don't want to miss out.
- In an affair, there is a "holiday" feeling, with romance, adventure, thrilling excitement, chemistry,

and intense intimacy. Some women like the aura of being a temptress and enjoy the feelings of illicit sex and secrecy.

- It is much easier to be a lover than to be a wife.
- Most married women do not want to hurt their partners; they try to protect them, and they try to avoid a scene or showdown.
- Most women do not want to break up their marriage if their affair is discovered, nor do they want their lover to get a divorce for them.
- Most women do not want to marry their lover; their antennae would be up, and they would suspect that the lover wouldn't be faithful to the marriage.
- In a recession there is a decrease in the number of divorces and an increase in the number of extramarital affairs.

Having an affair can have some positive long-term effects. The spouse may begin to look good when compared to an unstable, fickle lover. The cheating partner may feel guilty and may resolve to make amends, putting more energy into the marriage to make it work. That could include going for marriage counseling. But it is essential that all contact with the other woman (or man) must stop—immediately. A good book for couples who want to put their battered marriage back on track is *The Monogamy Myth: A Personal Handbook for Dealing with Affairs* by Peggy Vaughan (New York: Newmarket, 2003), rev. ed.

So, let's not throw out the baby with the bathwater. There is a good possibility that you and your wife can get your marriage back on track, but it's difficult without a skilled therapist to give you some guidance and help both of you relearn how to communicate with each other. While you are waiting for your appointment, do read the books, keep a journal, and start doing all the nice little things that show your partner how much you care, that you are committed to making the marriage work and that you still love her.

AFTER SEX

Dear Sue: How come guys are so dumb about women? My boyfriend and I have great sex—I am completely satisfied. But as soon as he rolls off me, he lights a cigarette, grunts, and promptly falls asleep. I'm wide-awake, wanting him to hold me for a while, and he's snoring. Thanks a lot, big guy. He says he can't help it, it's a man thing.

Sue says: Let's look at the difference between male and female expectations of sex. For most women, sex is equated with love. Before a woman has sex with a man for the first time, there are several magic statements that she really wants to hear: "I love you," "I need you," "I want you," "Babe, you are the greatest," and "I will never leave you." Guys know that—that's why they use those lines, because they work. But guys have trouble believing that after great sex (even so-so sex), many women need some nonsexual body contact, to be reassured that they are loved and appreciated. That means hugging, cuddling, snuggling, and nuzzling.

On the other hand, when a male is having sex, his endorphin level is very high, and almost immediately after ejaculation, he goes through a refractory phase in which he loses his erection and all his systems gear down. This phase is instantaneous, whereas females come down gradually.

Enter negotiation skills. You must be able to tell your partner what you need without putting him down and making him feel like an insensitive jerk. He needs to be able to explain why cuddling and hugging is difficult for him right then, and then you may have to compromise and make a deal. He will snuggle and cuddle for about five minutes and then fall asleep in your arms. Sounds good to me.

AGING AND SEX

One of the most pervasive myths today is that sex is the prerogative of the young and the coupled. They have a monopoly on it, and anybody who is over forty-five and without a partner might just as well forget it.

Truth is, you were sexual before you were born, and you will be sexual until the day you die. Your sexual drives, desires, and activities may change, but you are still sexual and capable of fully enjoying a wide variety of sexual behaviors. These include touching, hugging, holding, and kissing passionately. You can enjoy petting, fondling, genital stimulation either by yourself (solitary masturbation) or with a partner (mutual masturbation), oral-genital sexual contact, and use of a vibrator. These can be as pleasurable and satisfying as sexual intercourse and should not be seen as second best.

Dear Sue: What's a lady to do if she's a healthy seventy-year-old and there are no men around?

Sue says: This is a real problem. For every available male over sixty, there are eight females, because women live longer and are generally healthier. But you do have some options. You can give yourself permission and learn to masturbate, or you can develop a loving same-sex relationship. What have you got to lose?

I recently received a wonderful letter from a sixty-eight-year-old gentleman:

Dear Sue: *My wife is sixty, and we still enjoy being together and fooling around, but I do not get an erection that is hard enough for sex. If I "play with it," I get an erection, but it goes down very quickly. My wife seldom wants intercourse because she is so dry, and no amount of petting can make her wet. Sue, is our sex life relegated to the back burner for the rest of our lives?*

Sue says: Absolutely not—it has simply changed. That old urge to merge is reduced, but there is a lot more to sex than penis-in-vagina. Let's look at the aging process and the changes that happen to our bodies. Once you understand them, the pressure is off and you can relax and enjoy.

There are the obvious external body changes—gray hair, baldness, and the redistribution of body fat so that your broad, manly chest slips down to your belt line and you develop a "Molson muscle." Such medical conditions as hardening of the arteries make it more difficult for your heart to pump blood to all parts of your body, including your penis, and therefore it takes longer to get an erection. This erection may be less firm than when you were a younger man.

You may experience periodic impotency or erectile failure (the inability to attain or maintain an erection firm enough for vaginal penetration), or you may experience premature, or rapid, ejaculation (ejaculating before ten strokes or before three minutes of intercourse). Mature males frequently tell me that it doesn't shoot out anymore, it just drizzles. They no longer have that sense of urgency. Fear of failure or feeling inadequate may make them hesitate to "go for it."

After twenty-five years of marriage and sex with the same partner, there is bound to be some monotony: sexual activity becomes ritualistic; it always seems to happen on a Friday night after the news, in the missionary position, with the lights out. It is difficult to be exciting and innovative in your lovemaking with your partner if you haven't let loose lately, or ever.

In the past you might have been uncomfortable if you did not ejaculate every time. Now, that sense of urgency is reduced, so if you ejaculate, it's great, but if not, no problem. As long as you and your partner are happy with the duration of intercourse, it is not a problem. If it is a problem for you or your partner, do check with your family doctor and check out the possibility of Viagra or the newer medications for this sexual dysfunction.

Now let's take a look at what happens to a woman's sexuality as she ages. Females experience menopause and the cessation of menstruation anytime between the ages of forty-five to fifty-five. We all know about wrinkles and sagging breasts and mood swings and hot flashes. But there are other less obvious changes that directly affect sexual performance and pleasure.

Like older men, older women take longer to become sexually aroused. They also require more direct stimulation and experience less urgency to reach orgasm and little or no discomfort or dissatisfaction if they do not achieve it. Both males and females can reduce stress, anxiety, and performance pressure if they believe that they pleasured their partner as well as themselves.

There are definite changes in arousal patterns as we age. Inadequate lubrication can make sex painful for women and leaves them vulnerable to cystitis (bladder infections) and repeated or chronic vaginal infections, which cause considerable discomfort and leave them less than enthusiastic about sex. The mucous membranes that line walls of the vagina become thinner, drier, and more vulnerable to tears and vaginal infections. Use generous amounts of a commercial lubricant such as K-Y Jelly to relieve discomfort.

Some medications such as antidepressants, high-blood-pressure prescriptions, barbiturates, and some heart drugs can reduce sex drive. Do talk to your doctor about any medications you take and ask how they will affect sex drive.

These changes will be less noticeable in women who have been on hormone replacement therapy (HRT) after the onset of menopause. If a woman has not been taking hormones and using lubricant does not relieve the dryness, it's a good idea to explain the changes to the gynecologist and explore the possibility of HRT. Recent research shows that HRT can be recommended if menopausal symptoms are affecting your mental or physical health. They recommend short-term intervention with HRT until the symptoms subside. You could also request a hormone patch, or a hormone cream that is applied to the genitals every day.

There has been a great deal of publicity about women using Viagra, but it has not proved successful. Extensive new research has been conducted on testosterone replacement therapy (TRP) for women experiencing low sex drive. Ask your doctor.

Either you or your partner may be turned off if one of you has gained a great deal of weight, if you are not careful about personal hygiene, or if you are drinking heavily. It is difficult to fake interest when all you feel is disgust and contempt.

If your relationship is a stormy one in which there is anger and resentment, it will be difficult to turn hostility off and passion on. You may be hesitant to suggest that you see a counselor together to explore your feelings. In reality, many couples would benefit from some counseling about sexuality as they grow older. Once you begin to understand your feelings and have some awareness of why your partner reacts and responds as she does, the antagonism decreases and you become capable of greater intimacy, which generally leads to increased sexual pleasure.

Open, honest communication is the key to success in a loving relationship if it is to endure and be pleasurable. If the trust level is up, if the intimacy is there, it is easier to discuss what stimulates you and what is not pleasurable for you.

Go for the romantic stuff—candlelight, soft music, and even a sexy nightie. Spend time touching, hugging, holding, kissing, and caressing. Make use of things that turn you on, whether they be sexual fantasies, reading erotic literature, watching erotic videos together, or looking at *Playboy* and *Playgirl* magazine, unless your partner finds that unacceptable. Try to incorporate some sexual fantasies into your lovemaking. So if you have always wanted to do it in a rocking chair or on a blanket in front of the fireplace, or you want to play strip poker, cover your partner in whipping cream, or give a gentle spanking, why not try it? Be innovative, and above all, keep your sense of humor.

And don't forget—if your partner is not interested in sex right now, all is not lost. You are quite capable of self-stimulation to satisfy yourself—masturbation is not second best. For many people it is as satisfying as sex with a partner. You are not totally dependent on your partner. If you remove the performance pressure, you will be more relaxed. This is true of both males and females.

Sex is like riding a bicycle. Once you do it, you never forget, but you may be a bit slow and wobbly if you haven't done it for a long time. Remember, you can't do at eighty what you did at eighteen. But think about it—in all probability it wasn't that great at eighteen either.

The next letter is a classic example of the problems that can arise if you have not had a partner for a long time.

Dear Sue: *I'm sixty-five years old, and my wife died five years ago. Recently I met a wonderful lady. We hold hands, hug, and kiss, and I get the feeling that she would like to do more, but I am afraid to start for fear she will think I am a dirty old man.*

Sue says: A generation ago, people did not talk about sex, so I can understand that you may not have the words or be too embarrassed and shy to bring it up. You may have to think about what you want to say and even practice saying it so it does not sound like a foreign language.

It will be much easier if you say it in terms of how you feel, using "I" terms. You could start out by saying, "I find I really enjoy being with you. It just feels comfortable and natural. I am really beginning to care for you and I hope you feel the same way." At this point, she will probably reassure you that the feelings are mutual. If she does, carry on by saying something like, "I love kissing you, but I am a little embarrassed to go any further, so I thought I'd check it out with you." At this point, she can tell you how she feels. Maybe she believes sex belongs only within marriage. Maybe she is afraid you will compare her body to your wife's and won't like it. Maybe she never did enjoy sex and wants to avoid it. Maybe she will be enthusiastic.

But if you talk about it, you will know, and then you can decide what you want to do for the future of that relationship.

If you have not been involved in intercourse or even masturbation for a long time, you may find it difficult to jump-start your sex drive again. Although the myth "use it or lose it" is not true, it may take time and encouragement from a loving, caring partner. I hate to bring it up, but you must discuss Safer Sex, just in case either of you has herpes, warts, gonorrhea, or another STI, including HIV/AIDS. And you should also know that if you do have intercourse, or even heavy-duty petting, there is a chance that you could develop a bladder irritation or infection. Now, this is not a disease—it happens to most women who suddenly start having sex again. Don't be embarrassed or upset.

If you suspect you have a bladder infection, you should immediately get an appointment with your doctor and take an early-morning, midstream sample of urine. If it is cloudy, the doctor will send it to the lab and will probably give you a prescription for antibiotic pills. You must take the pills as prescribed, without going off them even if you think the infection is all cleared up, and abstain from sex until you are cured. The doctor may give you a prescription for pyridium pills if the burning sensation is severe. You need not worry if your urine turns as orange as a duck's foot when you are on this medication! And the doctor will likely tell you to drink lots of water. Cranberry juice helps, too. Finally, it's important for women—especially those who are susceptible to bladder infections—to urinate right after sex. In all probability, you will not get the infection again. (For more information, please see page 49 or check out *The Gynecological Sourcebook* by M. Sara Rosenthal [New York: McGraw-Hill, 2003] 4th ed.)

Enjoy. We call it honeymoon cystitis. Your friends will be jealous!

Dear Sue: *My sixty-year-old brother has always been very sensible, but he suddenly started going out with a thirty-two-year-*

old woman who has young children. What's he thinking? I think he should find somebody his own age.

Sue says: It sounds to me as though you definitely disapprove of your brother enjoying a relationship with a younger woman. Are you assuming he is experiencing a midlife crisis or is attempting to recapture his lost youth, and is living out a fantasy that is shared by many men—spectacular sex with a woman, no hassles, no expectations, and no recriminations?

Are you hoping this is just a fling, and if he gets it out of his system he will date women his own age? Are you wondering what she is getting out of the affair—love, companionship, prestige, or money—or do you feel that she is being used and she is a fool?

Could it be that you resent him enjoying young love at his age? Consider the reverse scenario. It's not a new phenomenon, but now they have given it a name: cougars, or older women who are out on the prowl to attract younger men. It may be simply for a one-night stand, or it may develop into a long-term relationship. In general these women are wildly enthusiastic about sex, have few inhibitions, and are very innovative. This does not endear them to the mothers or wives of males involved with cougars. Most women regard them as sluts or whores and express disgust at and contempt for their amoral behavior. These same wives and mothers may actually just be threatened or afraid that their son or partner may get involved with a "tramp" like that.

In reality, cougars are usually smart, mature women with good careers. They're sophisticated, have probably been married but are now separated or divorced, and do not want children. They like to be independent and in control, and they like feelings of power and dominance. When they want sex, they go out on the prowl—hence the name cougar.

Valerie Gibson, a Canadian, has written a great book, *Cougar* (Buffalo: Firefly Books, 2002). It's a fun and enlightening read.

As a caring, concerned sibling, would you take time to explore your reactions to your brother's new relationship? Are your objections truly valid? Could you discuss your reactions in a nonjudgmental way, then allow him to decide what is in his own best interest? Depending on the outcome, you may find you want to celebrate this newfound love with both of them.

AIDS

Dear Sue: There is so much confusing information about AIDS. Can you give us the straight goods?

Sue says: When we first became aware of AIDS in the 1980s, the publicity focused on pain and death and did not provide much accurate information except that we should practice Safer Sex. To explain how the virus is transmitted, we need to be explicit, sometimes using slang rather than "medicalese," which can be confusing.

AIDS is caused by the human immune deficiency virus, or HIV. It is a very weak virus that dies upon exposure to heat, cold, air, light, soap and water, rubbing alcohol, bleach, and all disinfectants.

The virus is very concentrated in some of the infected person's body fluids; for example, lubrication (pre-cum) or ejaculate from a male, breast milk, vaginal lubrication or menstrual blood, and blood from a cut or wound.

To infect you, one or more of these fluids must gain access to your body, through an open sore or cut, severe acne, or eczema. Recent research seems to indicate that the virus can pass through certain mucous membranes, even if there is no break in the surface. This makes oral-genital sex and unprotected sexual intercourse risky behavior.

Once the virus gets into your body, it multiplies rapidly, and as it does, you gradually develop antibodies to counteract it. It takes approximately thirteen weeks for your body to develop enough antibodies for an accurate blood test to diagnose the presence of the virus. A negative test is generally accurate, but if you are anxious and have "AFR.AIDS," check with your doctor about the advisability of periodic retesting. You may be infected without knowing it, and if you are sexually active and are not practicing Safer Sex, you can infect your partner. Although you have the virus in your system, you probably have no signs or symptoms, so you may not realize that you need a test. And even if you are tested shortly after exposure to the virus, the test would probably be negative because it takes up to thirteen weeks for the antibodies to the virus to show up in your blood test. When they do show up, you are HIV positive, but at this point you do not have AIDS.

But HIV starts to destroy your T-4 helper cells, and your immune system will be weakened. You will probably still appear fine, although you may not be hungry and may feel fatigued. When you are unable to fight common infections, you are vulnerable to a form of pneumonia, diarrhea, systemic yeast infections, and a type of skin cancer called Kaposi's sarcoma. As soon as you get one of these opportunistic infections, you are diagnosed with AIDS.

New treatments are being developed to prolong life, but they may be toxic and hard on the body, and each time another infection hits you, you become weaker and more vulnerable. As yet there is no cure.

There are many myths about HIV/AIDS, and one of them is that it is confined to the homosexual community. Until recently, in North America AIDS affected primarily gay males, but now more and more women are becoming infected with HIV by sexual partners who are involved in high-risk behaviors. And in Africa, as many women as men are infected with HIV.

Dear Sue: *How do you know if you have AIDS?*

Sue says: Here are some of the most common symptoms:

- Swollen glands in your neck, armpit, and groin, which remain swollen for weeks or months.
- Chronic diarrhea that does not respond to treatment and results in severe weight loss, about five or ten pounds a week, for weeks.
- A deep, persistent cough, which is an uncommon form of pneumonia that does not respond to usual treatment.
- Kaposi's sarcoma manifests itself as large, flat purple-black tumors that spread and grow. Other than surgery, there is no effective treatment.
- Occasionally an infected person may experience an outbreak of herpes zoster, a form of shingles usually around the rib cage, or anywhere on the body.

The signs and symptoms may be different for women. They may have heavier or irregular menstrual periods, severe cramps; intercourse may be painful and they may develop endometriosis. Many women with AIDS have severe systemic yeast infections that do not respond to treatment.

Okay, now that you have some bottom-line information, but just how do you get the virus? Well, you need to know that in an infected person the virus is present in all body secretions but is more concentrated in some than in others. The virus is present in tears, but in such small quantities that you would have to inject at least one quart of tears directly into your bloodstream to get enough to infect you.

How about nasal secretions? Although there may be a few viruses present, there are not enough to cause an infection. Saliva? No, once again, there are not enough viruses present. So kissing—yes, even deep French kissing—is safe. Phew!

Breast milk? Yes, the virus is fairly concentrated in the breast milk of women with HIV. But we do not know if babies get the virus from breast-feeding or if the virus transmits through the placental barrier, infecting them during pregnancy, and there is just a delay in the virus showing up in tests after birth. There is new and effective medication that can be prescribed to HIV-positive women who are pregnant.

Genital secretions are all loaded with the virus. Lubrication from the genitals of both males and females who are sexually aroused, vaginal secretions, menstrual blood, and male ejaculate all contain high concentrations of the virus. So any unprotected intercourse is risky.

When an infected male has unprotected sex with a female, she is vulnerable if she has the slightest cut, abrasion, or cervical erosion, venereal warts, or herpes lesion, or if she is menstruating. There is now some evidence that the virus can penetrate through the mucous membrane that lines the cervix. So, if there is even the remotest possibility that her partner might be infected, she must insist that he use a latex condom. Sex is not worth dying for.

If a male has unprotected sex with an infected female, he will be okay unless he has a little pimple, pustule, wart, herpes lesion, or abrasion on his penis. Then the virus can enter his body and he may become infected.

Their genitals are external, so guys generally know if they have a sore on their penis, but because women's genitals are internal, they may not be aware that anything is wrong. This is why you should always practice Safer Sex by using a latex condom. (For essential information about Safer Sex and condoms, read the section on condoms on page 71.)

Here's another common question:

Dear Sue: *Can you get AIDS from giving your partner a blow job (oral-genital sex)?*

Sue says: Now you know that the virus cannot penetrate intact skin, although recent reports seem to indicate the possibility that the virus can penetrate intact mucous membranes in the esophagus in the back of the throat. Oral-genital sex might be considered risky behavior, particularly if you have an open sore in your mouth. I am talking about cold sores, cracks at the corners of your mouth, cankers or gum boils, or if you have flossed or cleaned your teeth and made your gums bleed, if you had a tooth extracted or if you bit your lip. These are breaks in the mucous membrane through which the virus could gain access to your body. If in doubt, practice Safer Sex.

Dear Sue: *Can you get AIDS from sex "by the back door" (bum sex or anal sexual intercourse)?*

Sue says: Here are the facts so you can make informed decisions about your sexual behavior.

[23]

In anal sex, a male inserts his penis into the rectum of another person, whether male or female. Anal sex is classed as high-risk behavior for the transmission of all sexually transmitted infections (STIs), including HIV/AIDS, because the mucous membrane that lines the rectum is very thin and tears easily during intercourse. If the mucous membranes tear, the virus in his lubrication or ejaculation can enter your body. Not only do you risk getting HIV/AIDS, it is very possible that you might also get anal warts, herpes, or gonorrhea or syphilis. All of these may be quite painful and difficult to treat. And there is always the possibility that the tears in the rectum will become larger and turn into a fissure (a crack leading to the outside of your body), which could become infected and would be very difficult to treat. And you might develop hemorrhoids (for more information, see Anal Sex on page 26). I am giving you this information so that you know what is involved and you can decide whether this is the kind of sexual activity you want.

Now, if you do decide you want to engage in anal sex, then, knowing the risks, you *must* practice Safer Sex. You must use a condom and lots of lubrication, and you both should be very relaxed. When you attempt to insert your penis into your partner's rectum, you must be very, very gentle; your partner must consent; and you must have a clear understanding that if your partner says "stop," "whoa," "ouch," or "no," you must stop immediately. (The same goes for vaginal sex.)

Anal sex is high-risk behavior. You must really know and trust your partner. But how can you know the details of your partner's sexual history? You can't, not really. Perhaps they tried injecting street drugs just once, but that could mean they have HIV/AIDS. They may have experimented with anal intercourse, either with a man or a woman, without practicing

Safer Sex, so they could be infected. How do you know for sure? You don't, so don't risk it. Insist on Safer Sex or no sex.

Dear Sue: *Is it okay to have sex without a condom if your partner says he has been tested for AIDS and is all clear?*

Sue says: No. You see, we do not test for the virus, we test for antibodies to the virus. We have to wait at least thirteen weeks for the antibodies to develop before we can test for them, and then we get a fairly accurate result. So your partner would have had to have stopped having sex thirteen weeks ago and then be tested, and then wait another two weeks with no sex until the results came back. If they were negative and he or she had had sex in the past four months with no one but you (and you used a condom every time), the person would probably be okay, but it's still better to practice Safer Sex. This is your life we are talking about. Sex is not worth dying for.

The "Dear Sue" question boxes commonly contain the question "How do you get AIDS from shooting up?" You may not know what is involved in doing heavy-duty drugs, so I will explain. A few people in your school say they have some "good stuff" and are going to shoot up. Being curious, you go along to watch. Then someone says, "Come on, try it, don't be a chicken, it won't hurt, you'll get a real buzz." So you try it. Your friends have a syringe, needle, the drug, a bottle of tap water, a metal spoon, a lighter, and an old nylon stocking. They pour some water into the metal spoon, add some of the "good stuff," hold the lighter underneath, and heat the water to dissolve the powdered drug. Then they draw the solution up into the syringe, tie the nylon stocking around their arms, and watch the veins pop up. They run the needle parallel to the vein and angle it right in. To be sure it is in a vein, they draw back and some of their own blood goes into the barrel of the syringe. (There's no sense shooting it into the muscle or tissue—they won't get high but will get a humongous bruise.) Then they pass that needle to somebody else, and that person shoots up. If anyone in that "shooting gallery" has the AIDS virus, that residual blood in the syringe will be loaded with the virus, and if you shoot up using that syringe you will be injecting it directly into your bloodstream. You got it—doing drugs is the dumbest thing you can do.

Contact a local AIDS group for more information on clinic locations and needle-exchange programs in your area.

ANAL SEX

In her book *Hot and Bothered* (Toronto: Key Porter Books, 1992), Wendy Dennis said that today anal sex is what oral sex was thirty years ago. And judging by the calls and letters I get asking about anal sex, it does appear to be another taboo shot down in flames. While many people regard anal sex as abnormal and/or too gross, like it or not, anal sex is a fact of life, and we need information so that we understand the risks and can protect ourselves if we decide to try it.

Dear Sue: *My boyfriend wants to have sex "by the back door." I'm not sure I like the idea. Is it safe?*

Sue says: It sounds to me like you're looking for a way out of that back door. First, we need to be very clear what he is talking about, because sex "by the back door" can mean either anal sex or vaginal sex with the female in the doggie position (on her hands and knees). So do make sure you know exactly what he means.

Let's assume he is talking about anal sex. Basically, the rectum was not designed for penetration. The mucous membrane of the rectum is very thin and tears easily. Because it does not heal very fast, it is vulnerable to infections. Also, it can enlarge to a fissure or a crack leading to the outside of your body. These are painful and slow to heal. There is the remote possibility that a fistula (or canal) could open up, allowing feces to reroute into the abdominal cavity or into the vagina, which is likely to cause a bad infection and must be treated surgically. There is also the increased risk of hemorrhoids (protruding rectal veins), which are quite uncomfortable.

If you do decide to engage in anal sex, your boyfriend must use a latex condom and lots of non-oil-based lubricant (which won't weaken the condom) because anal sex is high risk behavior. I don't want to lecture here, but this is extremely important. If you and your partner do not practice Safer Sex, and if he is HIV positive and does not know it (this possibility always exists), then the virus will be present in his genital secretions and ejaculate, which makes you vulnerable to the virus. Only doing intravenous drugs with a nonsterile needle and syringe puts you at higher risk of getting HIV/AIDS than anal sex. But wait, there's more. You can get herpes or venereal warts around and inside your rectum, which are painful and difficult to treat, or syphilis or gonorrhea in the rectum treatable but not fun. (See *Gonorrhea* and *Syphilis*.)

If you've read the information above and you still want to try anal sex, you will have to be very, very relaxed and willing, even enthusiastic. Are you going to be comfortable with the possibility that you might let loose with a mighty fart, or that he might get your feces all over the condom on his penis?

There may be another fear lurking at the back of your mind. If he wants to do this, what other quirky ideas is he going to come up with for you to try? And if you do agree to try it "just once," what if he really likes it and wants it all the time? Will he tease you and accuse you of being boring and a prig if you say no to doing it again?

Let's say you agree to try anal sex but find it is painful. If he says, "Just relax, it will be okay once you get used to it," just reach around and grab him by the testicles and say, "Just relax, it won't hurt once you get used to it." I'm not trying to be funny here—he is causing pain and must stop immediately.

In all sexual activity, there must be no coercion, manipulation, threats, exploitation, or promises. So, if he says, "Do it for me," or, "It's the only way I get turned on," then you must admit he is not thinking of you at all—he is using you to get what he wants. This does not bode well for the future of this relationship and you might be well advised to get out of it now, because the next step could be physical coercion and violent assault. For more information about anal sex, read *Anal Pleasure and Health: A Guide for Men and Women* by Jack Morin, Ph.D. (San Francisco: Down There Press, 2000), 3rd rev. ed., or *The Ultimate Guide to Anal Sex for Women* by Tristan Taormino (San Francisco: Cleis, 1997). Think about it and decide for yourself. The following letter gives more advice if you do decide to try anal sex.

Dear Sue: *My wife and I watched an erotic video and we were both turned on by the anal sex and want to try it.*

Sue says: The key words here are "Gently, Bentley." There are a few bottom-line rules:

- Practice Safer Sex using a condom and lots of lubricant.
- Your partner must be very relaxed and willing.

- Agree ahead of time on a stop signal, such as "ouch," "quit," or "whoa," or even a firm "no," and you must agree to respect that command.
- Put a condom over your finger, lubricate it well, then slowly and gently insert one, then two fingers into your partner's rectum. When he or she is fully relaxed, put a condom on your penis and slowly insert it, a little at a time.
- Do not use force when thrusting, or you could cause damage.
- When you withdraw your penis from your partner's rectum, you must hold on to the condom so that it does not slip off and remain in there.

Being involved in anal sex is a very personal decision, and if you have good, accurate information, then you can make a rational decision based on fact and feelings. Anal sex is not confined to the homosexual community. Many heterosexual couples enjoy this activity. Usually it is at the suggestion of the male, who is curious and wants to experiment. Females who are comfortable with their appearance and enjoy innovative sexual activity may also find sex "by the back door" pleasurable. Just think, if you are in the doggie position he can manually stimulate your breasts and clitoris at the same time. Who knows? You may both really enjoy it.

Check out the new video from the Sinclair Intimacy Institute, *The Better Sex Guide to Anal Pleasure*, part of their Forbidden Pleasures Video Series. It's available at www. bettersex.com.

ANGER

As I see it, there are three major emotions: mad, glad, and sad. All others are feelings: disappointment, joy, rejection, and relief. Originally, anger was one of the Seven Deadly Sins, along with lust and slothfulness.

Of all the emotions, anger is the one we have the most difficulty dealing with. We have permission to express gladness or to feel happy. Society has limited tolerance for sadness, and there is some support for grieving and mourning for a short period of time, although very soon people start to think it's time to "get over it and get on with life." However, anger is not sanctioned by polite society.

Only now are we beginning to give people the skills to deal with anger instead of sitting on it, seething or snarling, kicking the cat, or otherwise taking it out on others and ourselves. Finally, we are learning conflict resolution and anger management.

Dear Sue: *Boy, do we have a problem! I am a fighter, and when I am angry, I want to get it out, but my husband internalizes his anger. He becomes remote and silent. While I am ranting, raving, and roaring, he just continues to do his own thing with me bellowing behind him. I get so frustrated, and things go nowhere.*

Sue says: Wrong. Things are going somewhere—straight downhill. He controls you with silence, and you fight back with a barrage of words. You may be rewarded with four days of the silent treatment, during which you don't look at each other or talk to each other. You would both probably benefit from taking a workshop on communication, learning how to talk to each other without a power struggle.

Your partner needs to learn that it is okay to have feelings and that it is safe to talk about them. Read and practice the section on communication on page 232. Use "I feel" language in statements such as, "When you do that, I feel angry and frustrated." If that does not get your partner's attention, then you can say, "I need you to listen to me, and I need to know you are hearing me." Then your partner can paraphrase what you are saying. If it is not a good time to settle the argument, arrange a time when you will not be interrupted, and keep that time available. You will probably be calmer, cooler, and more logical. But don't keep score. Saying "I gave in to you last time. You owe me on this one" is manipulation.

Also, learn to negotiate. If your life does not depend on it, then come to some agreement that is acceptable to both of you.

Finally, do not store anger and resentment like a garbage bag in the middle of the floor. One day, the bag will explode all over the floor! Cleaning up all that hostility is a daunting challenge.

Dear Sue: *My girlfriend is Irish, with red hair and a temper to match. I think she uses this as an excuse. What can I do?*

Sue says: Redheaded Irish certainly do not have a monopoly on bad tempers. But if as a child your girlfriend observed her parents throwing things and slamming doors, then monkey see, monkey do, she follows true to form. Her behavior is designed to intimidate you so that you drop the subject. She may be convinced that you won the last battle, and she's determined not to let you win again. Or she may feel threatened, fearing she does not have the power and control in the relationship. So she may resort to guts and gusto to win the day for her.

Does she feel that you are so logical and verbally adept that she will lose every fight unless she creates a scene to throw you off? Or, does she believe the best defense is a strong offense, so that she goes in with all guns blazing, hoping that you will be too tired to fight, or that you will simply decide it is not worth it and she will win the battle? Problem is, she will eventually lose the war if you feel overpowered and bail out. When your girlfriend is in a rage, say something like, "Obviously you are upset, and I will come back when you and I can talk about it," and walk away. When she has chilled out, you can say, "You were really upset this afternoon. Do you want to talk about it now?"

Or, you could say, "I have difficulty talking to you when you are angry. I don't know what to do other than to wait until you are calmer. But this scares me because I do not want to live my life trying to avoid your temper." Later, when she is calm, try: "Would you consider getting some counseling?" This counseling is called anger management.

You might want to read one of these books together and discuss your reactions: *The Dance of Anger* by Harriet Lerner, Ph.D. (New York: Quill, 1997), and *Don't Go Away Mad: How to Make Peace with Your Partner* by James Creighton, Ph.D. (New York: Doubleday, 1991).

Dear Sue: *We have the best sex after we have had a hoot 'n holler fight. Is this normal?*

Sue says: Why not? Your adrenaline is up, the juices are flowing, and you vent all that anger. Later, you both experience resolution, settlement, and a glorious reunion. My only concern is that along with those intense makeup sessions, you have tender, gentle, romantic times, too. Although balance and diversity add spice, what you describe could be part of a pattern of abuse, remorse, reconciliation, great sex, anger, and more abuse. Obviously, that would be a destructive cycle.

ANOREXIA

Dear Sue: *I am anorexic. Do I still have to use birth control? My boyfriend won't marry me until I gain some weight back, but at the rate I'm going, it may be a long time.*

Sue says: Women with anorexia are firmly convinced that they are obese, and that if they could only lose another five pounds they would look much better. We look at them and see a skeleton, but they see fat.

But anorexia is not something for which you can just say "eat up" and expect it to work. A mouthful is an ordeal for somebody who has this eating disorder, and if that person does manage to eat, there is always the temptation to barf it up or to take a laxative or exercise furiously to work it off.

The theory is that females do not menstruate or ovulate unless a certain proportion of their body weight is fat, but you certainly can't count on that. In third-world countries where much of the population is malnourished, the women manage to get pregnant and deliver small but normal babies. If it is important not to get pregnant at this stage of your life—and I would say that you should work on your health problems before you consider it—you should definitely use birth control.

Physically, there is no reason why you can't take the Pill. Some women find it makes them hungry and they gain weight. But your doctor may recommend a barrier method such as condom and foam, the sponge, or a diaphragm. A word of caution: if you gain or lose more than five pounds, you must ask you doctor to check the diaphragm to make sure it still covers your cervix.

It will take good, in-depth counseling over a long period of time for you to learn to accept your body and even like it. Eating disorders are frequently the outward manifestations of deeper personal problems resulting from childhood family conflict—your parents' unrealistic expectations of you, or perhaps some form of abuse. Threatening or bribing your partner will not work in the long term. Therapy will, so do start now. Good luck.

APHRODISIACS

Dear Sue: Is there anything I can give my girlfriend to make her horny?

Sue says: Young males may seem to be horny all the time, with nonstop erections from age twelve to twenty. But although we do not have any reliable statistics, most sex researchers believe that teenage females are sexually aroused more often than they care to admit.

Folks have been trying to find a love potion for generations, and perfumes are simply odors designed to increase desire. Recent research reveals that the smell of fresh perspiration is a turn-on. Yet we are too uncomfortable to accept the fact that genital odor is an aphrodisiac, and one of the main functions of pubic hair is to trap that scent. A few years ago, many genital deodorant sprays were advertised. Women who used them discovered that their genitals developed a nasty allergic reaction to the spray, and now they are not available. As long as you practice reasonable hygiene, taking a bath or shower every day, the distinctive smell of your genitals will be stimulating to your partner.

Teens have heard many stories about aphrodisiacs that are guaranteed to make her "hot"—things like peanut butter, oysters, or celery. In some countries, people continue to purchase ground rhinoceros horn, dried beaver testicles, or a mixture of ground crickets, spiders, and ants in honey. As interesting as these substances are, there's no truth to the claim that they increase sexual desire.

Requests for aphrodisiacs generally come from young males trying to turn their girlfriends into raving, insatiable nymphomaniacs. Women tend to rely on their feminine charms instead of Love Potion No. 9.

Truth is, there is no such thing as a nymphomaniac. There are some folks who like sex a whole lot, or use it to meet other needs, such as getting attention, love, excitement; fighting boredom; exerting power or control; or avoiding emotional intimacy. Also see *Sex Addiction*.

Dear Sue: *What is Spanish fly, and where can I get it?*

Sue says: This question really scares me. Spanish fly is a powder made from a beetle found in Europe, and if your girlfriend takes it internally, it will cause inflammation and irritation of the urinary tract, which could result in permanent damage to her urinary system. Spanish fly makes the blood vessels around a woman's genitals dilate and throb, itch and burn. This throbbing isn't a result of sexual arousal; it's caused by inflammation and irritation.

If you really care for your partner, you will not add this to her drink with hopes that she will become amorous. If you have to rely on that, you are in trouble.

Dear Sue: *I have heard that there is a new testosterone patch that will increase the sex drive of both males and females. Is this true?*

Sue says: The most frequently heard complaint by both males and females in any sex therapist's office would be, "We have a good relationship, but I'm just not interested in sex," or, "I'm just not turned on anymore." Low Sex Drive (LSD), or Inhibited Sexual Desire (ISD), is the most difficult problem to treat, usually involving months of intense joint counseling. It's expensive and not always successful.

Hormone replacement therapy for postmenopausal women was marginally effective in some, until a few doctors began prescribing a compound of estrogen cream and testosterone, applied to the genitals twice a day—and it worked.

About the same time, researchers were finding that as many mature males were complaining of LSD as women. Finally it dawned on them that males experience a type of "menopause," with many of the same symptoms as menopausal women: their testosterone levels drop, as well as their enthusiasm for life, love, and sex. This became known as "andropause."

Drug companies developed a testosterone patch called Androderm that's worn on a man's upper arm or buttocks and changed every week. Not only did men become more interested in sex, they were happier and had more energy and joie de vivre. Although not enough research has been done on the patch for women, some doctors are quietly prescribing it to their female patients.

Most recently, researchers have found that women who were not depressed responded well to the antidepressant drug Wellbutrin SR. This drug boosts the brain's production of dopamine, which is linked to sexual desire. After two weeks on the medication they reported increased interest and involvement in sexual activity.

If you or your partner (or both of you) is just not interested in sex but don't want to give up on lovemaking, do talk to your family doctor and find out what is available and what might be best for you.

What else do people to do try to increase sex drive? Such street drugs as marijuana do not make you randy, but in small quantities they do enhance sexual pleasure and decrease inhibitions. We do know that males who smoke four or more joints a week have a significant drop in testosterone, which reduces their sex drive and sperm count. Alcohol is still the most common substance used to lower inhibitions, and it seems to increase sex drive in both males and females. HIV/AIDS educators are concerned about people having casual sex while under the influence because they may be less discriminating in their choice of partners. They also might not practice Safer Sex, and thus risk exposure to the AIDS virus. Teens use liquor because they think it's cool, or to bolster their courage and provide them with an excuse, such as, "I was so drunk I didn't know what I was doing."

I have a major concern about abuse of alcohol. We all know that a little alcohol can make you relaxed and sociable, but drink just a little bit more and you may not be as careful in your choice of partners. Alcohol also lowers your inhibitions, so you may tend to do things you would not normally do. You may take chances, "just this once," and put yourself at risk for many diseases or an unplanned pregnancy. Doing soft drugs such as marijuana can have the same effect. So make it a rule—no casual sex while "under the influence."

Still, many, many couples find that a drink of wine to iron the wrinkles out of the day, to relax and mellow out, helps them share and become intimate with their partner and that it is enjoyable and increases desire.

The largest sex organ is between your two ears—daydreaming and fantasizing are really stimulating. And remember, the skin covering your whole body is one large erogenous zone, so do you really need drugs or alcohol to make you or your partner horny? Remember the old adage "One drink and you can do anything; three drinks and you can't do anything." It's impossible to have really great sex when you're numb. Popular women's and men's magazines always advertise "new" sex-enhancing pills. These are not drugs but a combination of herbs that are not approved by Health Canada or the American Food and Drug Administration. There is no reliable research to prove they are effective, and because there are no controls on the content or manufacture of these "pills," I would avoid them.

[b]

BATTERING: ABUSED MEN

Dear Sue: *Every now and then my wife beats the can off me. I want to know if this ever happens to other guys because I have never heard anybody talk about it, and I don't discuss it because I feel like such a loser. She hits me, punches me, and kicks me, once she threatened me with a knife. Other times she attacks me verbally. Have you ever heard of this before? Signed, Slugged.*

Sue says: The statistics on male partner battering are only starting to surface. The statistics are surprising—and we women do not like to acknowledge them. A University of Calgary study showed that 23.3 percent of women admitted to abusing their male partners, while 17.8 percent of husbands admitted to abusing their wives.

Battering women are more likely to use a weapon rather than physical force. And like you, "Slugged," males are reluctant to disclose the trauma or defend themselves. Many have been brought up to believe that a man does not hit a woman, so they simply take it. They may fear they will harm the weaker female, that she might escalate the attack, or that they might lose their cool and kill her. Knowing this, women continue their attacks.

So, "Slugged," now that you know you are not alone, here are some options for you:

- Call the police and file assault charges.
- Move out. Unfortunately, I do not know of a shelter for males.
- Get counseling for yourself, and conjoint relationship counseling if your partner is willing.
- Find a support group. Ask your therapist to help you locate one. You can contact an organization for abused women to ask about services for males.

Learning to Live Without Violence: A Handbook for Men by Daniel Jay Sonkin, Ph.D., and Michael Durphy, Ph.D. (Volcano Press, 1997), is a book you may find helpful. It is intended for men who batter women, but it also applies to women who abuse men.

BATTERING: ABUSED WOMEN

Dear Sue: *My boyfriend grabbed my arm and squeezed so hard that I had a huge bruise for two weeks. He said he was sorry and that it would never happen again. Should I believe him?*

Sue says: Although I do not like to tell people what they should or should not do, my immediate response is to end it—

fast. Some readers will insist he should have a second chance because he was only rough once, it's not like he hit you, and you may be losing the love of your life. Possible, but not probable. Statistics show that abusive patterns appear early in a relationship and are a clear indication that the abusive man feels powerless, has poor self-control, low self-concept and self-esteem, lacks communication and problem-solving skills, and probably comes from a family in which violence is acceptable.

There are other forms of abuse, including insults and put-downs, threats, faultfinding, and blaming you for things that are not your fault. An abusive partner may try to control finances so you are totally dependent on his handouts. As well, he may attempt to control your activities so that you are isolated from your family and friends.

Be aware that this kind of violence does not go away. It almost always escalates with time and as the abuser's frustration increases. Abusers will appear contrite, apologize, and promise that they will never hurt you again. But because they have never learned any other way to get what they want, when they are frustrated, they resort to what they know works for them—a smack, a punch, a kick, throwing you against a wall or down stairs or even using a lethal weapon.

Many men were taught to assert control over women, and those men who have witnessed battering or were abused themselves are most likely to repeat such violence. These men usually believe in rigid sex-role stereotypes and traditional roles for women and are more likely to resort to violence to enforce their rules. They are likely to be jealous and possessive, and feel threatened, particularly if their partner is respected at the office and popular with family, friends, or the community. A jealous partner will try to isolate his wife or girlfriend from these connections.

Abuse tends to escalate during a pregnancy, and abusive

males may target their partner's breasts, abdomen, or genitals, and in some cases even cause a miscarriage.

Women from abusive families often pick abusive partners. If a woman is abused once, she needs to know that regardless of how contrite her partner is, in all probability he will beat her again, and the battering may even escalate.

With that warning, if you are in an abusive relationship, find out in advance where shelters are located and whom to contact in an emergency. Keep an extra set of car keys and enough money for a fast getaway. Do open your own bank account and start saving for a "flee fund." Tell your family and friends what has been happening. This is not something you should be ashamed of, and you must not protect him. Write out the date, time, and circumstances that trigger each assault. Tell your kids that if they hear you scream, they are to phone 911 immediately.

When the cops arrive, press charges. Although you can drop the charges at a later date, counselors recommend that you let them stand until you are better able to decide what is best for you. And please do take advantage of counseling services that are available for both partners. This is the only way you can break the cycle.

There is no excuse for abuse and battering, but you can avoid the risk by calling it quits immediately. You deserve the best. He ain't it.

Dear Sue: I am married and have three kids. Whenever I have a few beers, I get out of control and I take it out on my wife. Last week I hit her so hard—actually, I kicked her so hard, I broke her ribs. She went to the hospital, and they charged me with assault. Now the police won't let me go near her or the kids.

Sue says: That's good, for you, for her, and for the kids. In all probability, you will have to go to court and you may have to go to jail. I hope you will become involved in Alcoholics Anonymous to help you stop drinking. I also hope the prison has mandatory counseling so that you can learn how to relate to others and how to deal with your anger in an acceptable manner. Some correctional centers offer individual guidance that will help you understand your need to dominate and control other people and your need for power in relationships.

You must begin to recognize that violence is your choice alone and that you are responsible for your anger. Your wife did not make you so mad that you lost it; you allowed yourself to lose it and you decided to act violently. That is the bottom line.

You must get into programs that will help you learn alternative ways of dealing with anger, conflict, and other emotions, and that will help you gain better self-concept and higher self-esteem. A good program will also help you establish trust so that you can be open and honest about your feelings and find nonaggressive ways to meet your needs. This treatment may take a long time and, depending on your personal motivation, may or may not be successful.

Before you and your wife even think of getting back together, you need marriage and family counseling. This is the first essential step to take if you hope to get your relationship back on track.

Statistics Canada has released the results of a study of 12,300 women aged eighteen to sixty across Canada. Findings were:

- 51 percent of Canadian women have been sexually abused.

- 48 percent were assaulted by someone they knew, not by a stranger.
- 29 percent of women were assaulted by their husband or partner.
- 63 percent of these women were attacked more than once. Usually they did not report the assault until it had happened at least ten times; some waited until it had happened up to thirty times.
- Violence breeds violence. Women who had a violent father-in-law were three times as likely to be victimized in their relationship.

Dear Sue: *I have difficulty understanding why women stay in abusive situations. I have talked to my female friends and we all agree that we would be out so fast . . .*

Sue says: Many battered women have disclosed that they had been victims of incest as children. It seems that women who were battered looked for a partner who was a rigid, traditional male, the sole breadwinner, head of the family, and confident. To many people this comes as a surprise, but research in Canada and the United States suggests that a male who fits this stereotype would be more inclined to be abusive. Women who have been victimized as children appear to accept this abuse.

There may be many other reasons why women stay in abusive relationships. They may not have the financial resources to leave, and think they lack marketable skills that would enable them to earn an income; they may be isolated and unaware that there are shelters for battered women and that they can get welfare. Their partner may have threatened to harm them if they leave. Many battered women may be terrified he will come and get them and kill them or the chil-

dren. They may feel other people will not believe their partner is abusing them because to the outside world he is a nice,
decent guy, involved in the church and community groups.
Women in these relationships may be determined to make
the marriage work, or feel bound by marriage vows—"for
better or for worse till death us do part."

Here are some more reasons:

- Women are taught to be peacemakers. They hope
  that their situation will get better, and they want to
  believe their partner when he says he is sorry, that it
  will never happen again. They are determined to forgive and forget.
- Some abusive partners may be quite charming and
  loving between periods of rage. Women want to believe that "this is the real man I married," so they
  make up a myriad excuses for his abominable behavior. "He was under stress," they may say to themselves. Or, "I should have kept the kids quiet so he
  could sleep."
- Some women have low self-concept and self-esteem
  and believe their partners when they say they are a
  "no-good piece of shit"; the women might not believe they deserve any better, that they are lucky to
  have someone. This may be reinforced by learned
  helplessness from early childhood if their mother
  was abused, and this learned behavior might be reinforced when their partner starts battering them.
- Some women are embarrassed to admit what is happening to them because it would mean they had
  been poor judges of character to love such a jerk.
- Some women have been raised to believe that you
  do not reveal nasty family secrets or "wash your

dirty linen in public" by charging a partner and taking him to court.

Your question is a little judgmental, as though you are so superior, it would never happen to you. This is victimizing the victim. What battered women need is our acceptance of their situation, and all our support to help them remake a decent, safe life for themselves and their children.

A book that might be helpful is *The Battered Woman Syndrome* by Lenore E. A. Walker (New York: Springer Publishing, 2000), 2nd ed.

BISEXUALITY

Dear Sue: My wife tells me that I have to "shit or get off the pot." We have been married for twelve years, have three great kids, and good jobs. Life should be good. Although I still enjoy sex with my wife, and I still fantasize about sex with women, I am enjoying frequent sex with another man. I told my wife, and we do practice Safer Sex. In the beginning we thought it was a phase I was going through and I'd get over it, but I still want both loves in my life. My wife is now convinced that I am becoming homosexual. Is there any hope for us?

Sue says: Yes, there is hope for you and your two loves, but it will not be easy. You may find that to make it work you will each need to have individual counseling and then together agree on a lifestyle that is acceptable to all three of you. A recent survey of eight hundred bisexuals in California showed that 20 percent had concurrent relationships. However, you may have to make a choice if your behavior is not acceptable to your wife or your lover.

I would be reluctant to label you as bisexual or homosexual. Research from the Kinsey Institute in 1984 claimed that 37 percent of males have had some same-sex experience. Would we classify those males as bisexual? Kinsey felt that occasional bisexuality is much more common than we realize. He devised a continuum, from zero to six, with zero as solely heterosexual and six as exclusively homosexual. Most people, men and women, fall somewhere in between. Other sociologists claim that, left to our own devices, without any negative sanctions being imposed by our society, we would all go through stages of being heterosexual, then homosexual, perhaps bisexual, and then we would have periods of celibacy. That is a scary thought for those of us brought up with rigid attitudes and values.

Many therapists agree that there are some differences between men and women who claim they are bisexual. They feel that men tend to stay with their marriage and have outside affairs. They seem to be able to separate the two aspects of their life into compartments. Almost 30 percent of males who classify themselves as "bi" live "in the closet" in a traditional marital family setting. They tend to be affluent and have jobs that allow travel and freedom.

Females tend to be less involved in sex with another female but have close intimate relationships with women. This emotional connection with another woman makes it difficult to remain married; they divorce or separate and the "bi" woman becomes involved in a lesbian relationship.

There is no definitive research that spells out exactly what bisexuality is. People cannot be rigidly categorized in that way. However, our society seems unable to accept ambiguity—it says you must be one or the other; you can't have it both ways and have the best of both worlds.

Bisexuals feel that they are between a rock and a hard place. They are neither fish nor fowl. They are not accepted in the straight community, and yet the lesbian and gay communities are not supportive of them. Unfortunately, there are few resources, support groups, or good books for bisexuals. An older book is *Bisexuality: A Reader and Sourcebook* by Thomas Geller (New York: Times Change Press, 1990).

Now that you have a general picture, let's get back to your situation. As you can see, labeling yourself as bisexual could make things difficult. Sexual attraction is never static; it fluctuates. You may need a good therapist to help explore your sexual fantasies, emotional, social, and sexual preferences. You need to examine how you identify yourself and your involvement in the heterosexual and homosexual communities.

After counseling, you may decide you are more comfortable with a label after all, that your preferences lead strongly in one way or the other. If so, keep in mind some of the reactions you may receive when you disclose a new or different sexual preference.

Some people insist that bisexuality does not exist, that it is simply a transition phase—the person is really homosexual and in the process of changing over. Or, they are experimenting, "trying it on for size."

Other people say you are selfish and inconsiderate because you are hurting other people. Still another point of view sees bisexuals as amoral and unstable or perverted. Some people ostracize bisexuals, blaming them for the spread of HIV/AIDS and other STIs.

Your partner's reactions will likely include:

- I can't deal with this.
- I can't fight this other sex partner. I can't win.
- How could I be so stupid? How could I miss knowing?
- What does that make me—unattractive, neuter, asexual?

- How will the kids react, our family and friends?
- How could you do this to me?
- Did he infect me with AIDS or STIs?
- Is this congenital—will the kids be "bi," lesbian, or gay?

A person does not consciously decide on sexual attractions; they just happen. Bisexual people who are unsure, confused, and anxious about their sexuality and who are rejected by their family and peers often withdraw, become secretive, and avoid others. Getting help becomes more and more difficult.

One hopes that society will begin to accept that bisexuals have erotic, affectionate, and friendly feelings for both males and females. Like most responsible adults, many of them are selective and choose their partners consciously. They are aware of the effects of their lifestyle on others, and try to reduce, if not eliminate, emotional trauma for others.

I like this wonderful statement: "There are more kinds of love than stars in the Milky Way."

Most lesbian and gay organizations now include bisexuals in their mandate. I can also recommend these books: *The Other Side of the Closet* by Amity Pierce Buxton (New York: Wiley, 1994); *Bi Any Other Name* edited by Loraine Hutchins and Lani Kaahumanu (Boston: Alyson, 1991); *The Bisexual Spouse* edited by Ivan Hill (New York: HarperCollins, 1989).

BLADDER INFECTION

Dear Sue: I know this is not really a sex question, but I am a widow and have not had a sex partner for a few years. Recently I have been seeing a gentleman, and we had sex. That was all right, but I got a bladder infection two days later. I was so embarrassed going to my doctor, but I got a prescription for antibiotics and I'm still on them. Do you think my partner has a disease? This happened on my honeymoon, too.

Sue says: We call this "honeymoon cystitis." If you have not had sex in a while, when you start again, all those ordinary bacteria that your body has not been exposed to for a few years suddenly are deposited on your genitals. The friction of penis-in-vagina intercourse may irritate your urethra, leaving it vulnerable to the bacteria. Also, when you are sexually aroused, there is a "pulling up and in" motion of your genitals, and some specialists are convinced that some of these bacteria get sucked up into your urethra, and then into your bladder. Voilà, you have cystitis.

Although cystitis is a reaction to sex for men and women, it is not a sexually transmitted disease. Your partner does not need to see the doctor unless he has symptoms. You need never be too embarrassed to see your doctor. This person should not, and probably will not, pass judgment on you—that is not a doctor's role. If left untreated, cystitis can become chronic and very difficult to treat. Ignoring a bladder infection may do serious damage to your urinary system. You were right to get it checked out and to follow treatment prescribed by your doctor.

How do you know if you've got cystitis? Signs and symptoms include having a frequent and overpowering urge to urinate. When you do "go," often you are only able to produce two squirts and a dribble, that's it! And doing so does nothing to relieve the feeling of pressure in your bladder. And oh—it burns and hurts while you pee. You may have a low-grade fever, feel sluggish, or have a heavy sensation in your groin. Urine may be cloudy; if you collect a specimen of urine in a little glass bottle and let it sit, you may see sediment settled at the bottom.

Make an appointment with your friendly family doctor, and take with you an early-morning midstream sample of urine. The doctor will send it to the lab to see which bacteria is causing the infection and which antibiotic will work best.

In the meantime, you may be given a prescription for about forty sulfa pills. The doctor will likely tell you to drink gallons of water because sulfa can cause kidney stones, so you need to keep flushing it out. Drink lots of cranberry juice, and do take all the pills, even if the infection appears to have cleared up. It may flare up again if you don't follow instructions. If the burning sensation is severe, ask your doctor for a prescription for pyridium, a stronger medication.

A useful source of information on sex related illnesses is *The Gynecological Sourcebook* by M. Sara Rosenthal (New York: McGraw-Hill, 2003), 4th ed.

BONDAGE AND DISCIPLINE

Dear Sue: What is B&D? We were wondering what it involves.

Sue says: B&D means bondage and discipline. Generally the two go together, although each may be done separately. Bondage involves tying up a willing partner and stimulating that person by gently spanking him, kissing him, tickling with a feather, or other arousal techniques until he begs for mercy. Other arousal techniques can be used as well. For the submissive partner, the thrill and excitement come from a sense of being totally powerless and not being able to escape or control the situation. The other partner enjoys the sense of feeling dominant and all-powerful. Discipline usually involves spanking, pinching, biting, sucking, and pulling hair. These acts all involve inflicting pain on a willing partner who agrees to these activities.

The operative words here are "willing partner" and "agrees." There must be voluntary consent by both partners, with no manipulation or coercion.

If this is something you want to try, you both must establish some ground rules about how far you can go and agree on the words you will use to mean "stop now." Those who engage in bondage and discipline recommend you do not use words like "quit," "whoa," "ouch," or "no more" because they may be interpreted as signs of pleasure. Find another word, for example, "boat," "blue" "sky," or "mirror," words that have nothing to do with the activity.

If you use sex toys such as vibrators, dildos, or whips, you must practice Safer Sex. You want to get turned on, but you do not want to die of AIDS.

BOREDOM

Dear Sue: I have done everything I can think of to spice up a boring sex life. We are talking serious black nightie, romantic dinners with candlelight and wine, soft music to set the mood. Sure, it works, we have sex, but it is so monotonous and predictable that it is not worth it. We have never discussed it, but I suspect he feels the same letdown. What's to do?

Sue says: Let's be honest. The earth is *not* going to move every time you have sex, and not every meal is going to be a gourmet delight—once in a while you have to eat at a hamburger joint. But we all know there are ways to add interest to hamburgers. So it is with sex.

Rather than sex every Friday after the news with the lights

out, in the missionary position—or even after a fancy dinner in a black nightie—be innovative. Have fun and giggle. He could come out of the bathroom with a fig leaf that barely covers his erect penis, singing, "I Got You Babe" or "Sex, Sex, Let's Talk About Sex." You could dress up as a hooker in a tight short skirt and a little skimpy top and do a flirtatious bump and grind just for the fun of it.

Try different locations. The shower may be different, but how about the rocking chair, on top of the washer and dryer in spin cycle? No end to your imagination.

You and your partner could spend some fun time sharing and writing down your favorite sexual fantasies, some wild, some weird, some wonderful. Then you could take turns. He could make your fantasy reality. This could be sex on a bearskin rug in front of a fireplace after sharing a glass of wine. Then it's your turn to indulge his fantasy—sex in a sleeping bag on the balcony of your apartment with soft music and candlelight.

Erotic videos are very effective and can be great triggers for developing your own new fantasies. Then, there's always the *Kamasutra*, an ancient but still very popular book depicting numerous, almost impossible, but fun to try sexual positions.

BREAKING UP

Dear Sue: *My wife just up and left me. I came home from work to find she had taken about half the furniture, her car, and had left a note saying, "Sorry." What did I do?*

Sue says: The question "What did I do?" makes me suspect that communication between you and your wife was not open and honest. If it had been, you would have had some idea that she was unhappy, discontented, and wanted out. Her move did not happen suddenly one afternoon over tea. She thought about it, planned it, found a place to stay, knew exactly what she wanted to take, ordered a van or a friend with a truck, and made her move.

In all probability, signs and symptoms pointed to the fact that there was trouble in paradise. You may have had a vague sense that your wife was pulling away, distancing herself, and was less involved in the household and family. You probably ignored it or decided it was just a stage that she'd get over, blaming it on PMS, depression, stress, or overwork.

You may have been aware that she had new friends, new activities. If so, you may even have encouraged her because that took pressure off you. Meanwhile, she was developing a support system for herself.

There is a distinct pattern when a relationship starts to come apart at the seams, and you can identify it in retrospect. In the beginning a partner becomes angry and resentful, moody, argumentative, nitpicking, and faultfinding. Suddenly that changes. She becomes quiet, withdrawn, just turns her back and walks away. She won't look you in the eye. If you go near her, she quickly escapes. She may avoid sex by going to bed early and getting up early, or by sleeping on the sofa.

She still does her usual chores but she stops doing the nice little things, such as renting a movie you've wanted to see, or making your favorite dessert, or leaving a love note in your briefcase. By now, you are starting to be suspicious and concerned. You may ask, "What's wrong?" only to hear, "Nothing." Basically, by this point, she has made her decision. All that remains is to implement it.

At this point, you may suggest marriage counseling. If she agrees to go, it will probably be so she can say she tried. The damage has been done, and without knowing it, you are into a panic mode. The more you pursue the topic, the more she withdraws. A good counselor will recognize this and instigate mediation and separation counseling as a kind of damage control.

Even though you have separated, it is still not too late. Would you consider going for joint relationship counseling? A good counselor can help you both articulate your feelings and learn to communicate with each other. By now your wife probably has her own apartment, so she will have her own space and freedom. This makes it easier for her to decide if she wants to live alone permanently. If your relationship improves, she may wish to return and try again.

Don't mess up now. If you backslide into your old behavior and communication patterns, your relationship will be history.

If she refuses counseling altogether, and her departure is final, you will need help coping with feelings of failure and abandonment. You will go through the grieving process—denial, anger, trying to compromise and make a deal, depression, and finally acceptance. Until you reach that final stage, please continue to go for counseling. Otherwise, you will become one of the walking wounded.

Dear Sue: *I met this man who is just getting out of his marriage. There are two kids, he has weekend visitation, and I am just not too sure how I feel about getting involved with him.*

Sue says: Smart lady. Psychologists will tell you that we need a two-year healing period at the end of a relationship before we are ready to get involved in another.

The first year he will have intense feelings of anger, failure, rejection, loneliness, and recrimination at himself and toward his partner. This is a normal and necessary part of the healing process. He will have to do this work sooner or later, with or without you in his life; he'd better do it now and get it behind him.

The first year will also be one of anniversaries, his first holidays without her and his children. He has the memories of Thanksgiving turkey with the family. Christmas Day comes, and with it, issues of sharing the kids. Then he feels suddenly alone without her on Valentine's Day, Easter, and birthdays. By finding another partner immediately, chances are he simply postpones this essential but painful process.

He needs the second year to calmly and rationally analyze his marriage, identify and accept his contribution to the breakup, reestablish himself with his kids on his own terms, and get his life back on track. If he has another lady on the scene (i.e., you), she may be tempted to smooth things over and make it easy for him to avoid this essential area of growth. Without accepting his responsibility for the demise of the marriage, he will slip back into the old patterns that led to its breakup.

From your perspective, you are attracted to him and enjoy his company. Because women are taught to be nurturers and rescuers, you may get hooked into the savior role and end up planning activities for his weekends with the kids instead of letting him do it. You may protect him from loneliness and even become his surrogate therapist.

Many women in this situation are reluctant to keep a low profile in a man's life for those two years because they fear that some other lady will leap in and fill the gap.

If you are not willing to put the relationship on hold, then please do not try to become the be-all and end-all for him. Allow him the time and space to do the healing work that he must do. Try to explain this to him. He may not like it, but it will improve your chances of making a loving relationship work.

Dear Sue: *Is it possible to be friends with your ex? My husband and I separated after a long marriage and three grown children, and we have no hateful feelings toward each other. Friends don't believe it is possible. They insist it's temporary, that we will get back together again. Others say we should have a clean break.*

Sue says: I am hearing this from more and more couples who have split without rancor or resentment. No reason why you can't be together for the old family rituals, Christmas, birthdays, and the children's special events, and for problem solving. You have a history together and you can't simply put that behind you. Why should you be enemies? You may still care for your ex, yes, even love him platonically.

This may all be true, but problems will arise if one of you develops a new relationship. In all probability that person will have difficulty accepting your role in your ex's life, especially if you and he continue to plan family rituals together. Even if the new partner is included in these plans, he or she may feel like an "extra." A new partner would feel threatened and fearful that you will get back together with your ex. It would be wonderful if your new love could see your ex as your brother, as someone who is safe, neutral, harmless, and perhaps even fun to have around. But that takes a strong self-image and high self-esteem. You can only hope.

Dear Sue: *I was with my boyfriend for five years but it was kind of coming apart for a long time. Suddenly he met some blond bimbo, started acting like a jerk, and he left . . . after five years.*

Sue says: Your anger is just snapping through your letter. I'd guess you are flooded with a range of feelings. You feel relief—no more waiting for the other shoe to drop—and thankful that *you* did not have to end it. And you feel anger—how could he do this to you after five years of togetherness, whether it was good, bad, or indifferent? You are probably sad because it is the end of an era, and you may feel lonely because evenings at home are suddenly empty and silent. You may feel embarrassed when you are with your friends because he dumped you for a "bimbo," as you put it.

The scenario is so familiar. Usually the "breakor" (the person who initiates the breakup) will not initiate a move until somebody else is on the horizon. So a breakup does not suddenly just happen. It has usually been in the works for a while. The "breakee" (the person who is left) usually suffers more and for a longer period of time. Women suffer more either way, but men are more liable to keep the flame of love burning for a longer period of time.

That aside, you need to find coping skills for the next six months. My usual suggestions include:

- Feel free to cry, rant, rage, and roar for a while. You will find that the anger and pain do not last as long if you vent your feelings to friends and family.
- Allow yourself to go through all the old memories as they come up, that special gift, the clothes he liked you to wear. Put that photo in an album, cook his favorite dishes, and savor each bite thinking about what he is missing. Prepare all your old favorite meals, the liver and onions that he would not eat.
- Keep a journal of your thoughts and feelings. If you want to write a scathing or sentimental letter, do so, but do not mail it for at least six months. Wait to see

if you have healed and still feel this way. If not, you won't mail it. If so, you may need counseling. Renew all your old acquaintances and make new ones. Do this not with an eye to finding new love, but to enjoy different company. Take up old familiar sports, such as skiing, but also try something new, like windsurfing. If you lived together, put all his stuff away (you can haul it out later if you wish). Clean house like mad—redecorate or move furniture. Exercise regularly. Walk, follow a TV fitness class, or join a health club, bicycle, or swim. Eat well, but don't eat to fill an aching void. And do get enough rest. Be with your family for support.

Don't think, "We can still be friends." No, not yet. You need to get over the relationship. In reality, trying to be friends indicates that you are keeping the door open, trying to get a foot in, just in case you can get back together again.

In the beginning you will think about your ex all the time, but gradually you will find that you have not thought about him for over an hour. Eventually, he will not be the first thing on your mind in the morning or the last thing at night. Now you are healing. Keep on trucking.

Take time to examine what went wrong, what your role was in the disintegration of the relationship, if you could have rectified it, and how. List all the essentials for having a great relationship next time, because there will be a next time. And don't settle for less than the best.

Here are some great books on the subject: *Coming Apart: Why Relationships End and How to Live Through the Ending of Yours* by Daphne Rose Kingma (Conari Press, 2000), rev. ed.; *On Your Own Again* by Keith Anderson, M.D., and Roy MacSkimming (Toronto: McClelland & Stewart, 1992). *Uncou-*

pling: Turning Points in Intimate Relationships by Diane Vaughan (Vintage, 1990).

BREASTS, FEMALE

Dear Sue: They keep telling us to do breast self-examination. Fine, but my breasts feel like a bag full of marbles. My doctor calls them ropy breasts. Now isn't that a pretty picture? My boyfriend does not mind them, but cancer scares me.

Sue says: Ropy, or cystic, breasts are not unsightly, but the constantly changing cysts make monitoring more difficult because it is hard to identify new and different lumps and bumps. Do continue BSE (breast self-examination) to monitor changes and inform your doctor if there is a history of cancer in your family. If these concerns become an overriding preoccupation, have your doctor examine your breasts every six months. Although routine mammograms for women under fifty are not necessary, your doctor may recommend one if he considers you to be high risk.

A person does not automatically inherit cancer, but a tendency or a susceptibility to developing cancer appears to be hereditary. We all have cancer cells in our bodies, but most of the time our immune system keeps them in check. People with a family history of cancer are more vulnerable, so you need to find out who had what, when, where, and how it was treated. This is information your doctor needs.

Some research indicates an increase in cancer in women who have a diet high in fat and low in fiber, and that stress may be a contributing factor. Most recent research indicates that regular exercise reduces the risk of breast cancer in women in the thirty to forty-five age range. And I strongly recommend that you do not smoke.

BREASTS, MALE

Dear Sue: *Being a male, having noticeable breasts is not one of my goals. And mine are obvious—like, I'm bigger than my girlfriend. Is there surgery to reduce my bodacious "ta-tas"?*

Sue says: For a guy, having large breasts is equated with being femme, weak, and a wimp. The truth is, it is hereditary. Somewhere in your genetic pool your body size and shape was dictated, and "what you see is what you get." Also, you may be producing too much prolactin, a female hormone. I know, that's a shocker. Males do have small amounts of female hormones and females have small amounts of male hormones. That is what makes us androgynous, and gives us all that marvelous mix of maleness and femaleness.

If this is a major concern in your life, go to your family doctor and get it checked. You may be referred to an endocrinologist (hormone specialist) for a blood test to indicate prolactin levels.

If the test is normal, you might consider losing weight. Much mammary tissue is fat. And the doctor may discuss breast reduction surgery. This surgery may leave a circular band of scar tissue that may be more disfiguring than the large breasts, and there may be some reduction in erotic sensation around your nipples.

[c]

CELIBACY

Technically speaking, celibacy means abstaining from any form of sexual stimulation, either by yourself or with a partner. A person who chooses not to have sex with another partner, but practices solitary masturbation, is said to be partially celibate.

Priests and nuns take vows of celibacy so that they can devote all their energy and love to God. Some people, both men and women, go through periods when they voluntarily abstain from sex for a number of reasons: they are not in a loving relationship or their relationship is unstable; they may be fearful of diseases or unplanned pregnancy; they may be ill, exhausted, or under stress; or they may have an aversion to sex because of assault or sexual abuse in the past.

Dear Sue: I was happily married for twenty years and then we just grew apart—no sex, no intimacy for the next ten years. I moved out on my own, met a man, and had uproarious, drop-dead sex. I broke up with him because I felt all we had going for us was sex. I thought I would miss it terribly. I haven't. It has been eight years and I am just fine, thank you. I am responsible for my own sexual satisfaction, I have a great job, and I manage very well. My friends and family are all great huggers and cuddlers, so I am not missing body contact. I'm not into casual sex and I simply do not want a partner. Others think this is strange. Any insight?

Sue says: I am sure some therapists would say either you are rationalizing to explain your situation, or sublimating, burying and denying your real feelings. To me, it sounds as though you have found a nice balance between your work, your social life, and involvement with your family. A partner and a sexual relationship rank zip in your order of priorities. The problem seems to be what other people think. As a thoughtful and aware adult, you have to decide how much you are going to let other people determine what you do and how you feel. No matter what your age, as Rollo May said, "The unexamined life is no life at all." Personal growth never stops.

Dear Sue: *I have a very full life with my wife and family, and I just need to put sex on the back burner for a while. It's not that I don't like it, or am having an affair or punishing my wife by withholding sex. I just feel scattered, spread thin. My wife just cannot understand this and is really upset. Is this unusual?*

Sue says: No part of this problem is unusual. You may be feeling that you just need time to become more self-sufficient and at peace with yourself. Part of it may be a result of stress or passage into a new stage of life. That does not mean the way you feel is permanent, nor should your wife blame herself, you, the relationship, or your work. There is no explanation, it just is. She may not be missing the sex, per se, but the intimacy, the body contact. Are you still affectionate with your wife? If not, her reaction may soften considerably if you cuddle and snuggle with her every night before you go to sleep, again when you wake up in the morning, in front of the refrigerator—for the heck of it—before you leave for work, and after you get home. You get the picture. Many women equate sex with love. Show her you love her in other ways. This could greatly improve your situation.

Otherwise, I have a sense of two ships passing in the night. Neither of you is able to explain or understand the other's feelings. Two, maybe three sessions with a good marriage counselor could give you both some insight and reduce the anxiety, fear, and anger resulting from your desire to abstain from sex.

CIRCUMCISION, FEMALE

Female circumcision has received a great deal of publicity recently. You may find this next series of letters disturbing.

Dear Sue: I am so scared and I do not know where to go. I am a refugee from a country that practices female circumcision. Because all other women in my country had been circumcised as young girls, we thought the pain and the infections were a normal part of being a woman. Now that I am here I realize that what I had to endure was not necessary. I am married and pregnant. I was referred to a prominent female obstetrician who said that she would automatically do a cesarean section at the time of delivery. Is this necessary? In my country, women have babies more or less the normal way, even with circumcision.

Sue says: Before I answer this question, readers will need some information so they will know what I am talking about. Although this ritual is not a commandment in the Koran, Muslim women in many North African countries undergo a procedure we call female circumcision.

There are two types of circumcision. One is to cut out the clitoris. This technique effectively prevents most women from enjoying sex and reaching orgasm. Although we are aghast at the thought of this procedure, this is the less invasive one with fewer negative side effects.

The second is called infibulation. A girl's clitoris is removed, and the inside of the labia majora (large lips) are scraped raw with a sharp stick or a piece of bone. A hollow reed is inserted into her urethra so that the wound heals with a hole to allow for urination, and the labia are then sewn together, leaving a small opening for urine and menstrual blood. This is always done before puberty starts, usually around age nine, and without any anesthetic it is torture. Although the labia heal together, the girl is left vulnerable to infections, including bladder infections. Many female children die as a result of this procedure, and many more are afflicted for life. The "purpose" of this practice is to ensure a woman's chastity at the time of her marriage.

After a girl is married and when she first has sex, her husband literally tears the labia apart so the penis can enter the vagina. Her screams prove to the village that she is a virgin and he is a man. When she gets pregnant, the labia are cut apart to deliver the baby, and then sewn up again after delivery.

Societies in which this ritual is practiced hold that it guarantees wives will be faithful to their husbands. It also controls a woman's sexuality, which, if allowed to go unfettered, would lead to the downfall of society.

Fortunately, female circumcision is illegal in Western nations. Although we cannot change other people's religion and culture, we can provide education so that immigrants understand that they do not need to force their young girls to undergo this gruesome practice.

Now, to answer your question, it will take some research for you to find a doctor or obstetrician who would deliver your baby vaginally. The doctor will provide routine good prenatal care. When you go into labor the doctor will wait until your cervix is fully dilated (opened up). When you are bearing down, and the baby's head is right down on your perineum (genital area), you will be given a spinal anesthetic so that your doctor can surgically separate the labia, possibly do an episiotomy (small incision to widen the vaginal opening), and deliver the baby.

Now comes the big decision. In your country, some males insist that their wife have the labia sewn together again to make it tight for their sexual pleasure. After all your negative experiences with infibulation, you'll have to decide whether you are willing to have your labia sutured together again, or whether you will allow them to heal as normally as possible. And if your baby is a little girl, you must decide whether you would want this genital mutilation forced on her. Though this procedure is illegal here, we do know that it is being done by other women in your community, under nonsterile conditions, without anesthetic, and perhaps with serious long-term effects.

Networking with other women from the same culture may help you locate a good, supportive doctor or counselor. Most major centers have an immigrant women's health service where you can go for help. You can also contact your local department of public health for assistance.

We have an obligation to make information available to new immigrants, and offer services to raise consciousness and awareness that this mutilation does not contribute to women's health, happiness, or productivity.

CIRCUMCISION, MALE

It constantly amazes me that so many males have questions about circumcision. All this angst about a little piece of skin. (Then again, consider the angst about another little piece of skin, the hymen. Oh well.) This letter gives you some idea of the concerns folks have.

Dear Sue: I am expecting a baby, and I hope it is a girl because my husband and I simply cannot agree on whether to circumcise the baby if it's a boy. His parents are from Europe, where it is not done, and mine from the United States, where it is always done. What a fight. Poor little guy.

Sue says: Circumcision is a simple surgical procedure, usually done about three days after a baby boy is born. Generally, no anesthetics or painkillers are used, although some doctors are now using a topical anesthetic. The foreskin, or little piece of tissue that slides down and covers the head of the penis, is simply cut off with a scalpel. Then a piece of Vaseline-soaked gauze is wrapped around the penis, which becomes very swollen and sore. Urinating hurts the little guy for about three days.

In some cultures, circumcision is part of a religious ceremony. In North America, it is supposedly done for hygienic reasons, although many doctors feel it is merely cosmetic, and unnecessary. Some research seems to indicate that women whose partners have not been circumcised may be more prone to cancer of the cervix. It is believed this may be a reaction to smegma, that thick white waxy substance that collects under the foreskin if a male does not retract the foreskin and wash regularly with soap and water. (There are many factors that contribute to cervical cancer. We do know that the younger a female is when she starts having sex, and the more sexual partners she has had, the higher her chances are of getting cancer of the cervix. The risk is further increased if she has had venereal warts or if she smokes.)

A new study found that circumcised males were less vulnerable to AIDS. Researchers believe that the virus incubates under the foreskin (warm, damp, and dark) until there is a break in the mucous membrane. Then the virus gains access to the body. The "risks" associated with circumcision are largely a question of hygiene.

There is always the concern that if a little boy is not circumcised and his father was, the child will feel he is different, or not normal like Daddy. However, both parents can reassure the little guy that when Daddy was a baby, all little boys were circumcised routinely, but nowadays we know it is not necessary and both parents wanted to save their precious son that pain as an infant.

Some people, such as the man who wrote the following letter, regard circumcision as genital mutilation.

Dear Sue: *I am so angry and resentful at my parents. When I was born, they decided to have me circumcised. They chose to allow genital mutilation, without my permission. I resent them* *for making that decision without asking me. Is there anything I can do to get a foreskin back again?*

Sue says: Two components to this problem, the physical and the psychological, give it the double-whammy punch. Medically, yes, a skilled plastic surgeon could do a skin graft from tissue on the inner side of your leg. It is a complicated, three-stage surgery that is painful, and urinating becomes a problem for about three weeks; then there is always the risk of infection. For this reason, most surgeons hesitate to perform the surgery. Because it is considered cosmetic, it is not covered by medical insurance, and it is very, very expensive.

A good doctor would help you determine whether the lack of a foreskin is really the problem or if it has become the focal point for other feelings of resentment you have toward your parents. A good doctor would also tell you that having a new foreskin (especially a "fake" one) would not improve your quality of life or make you a better lover.

I would suggest that you take the money you might have used for surgery and invest it in good counseling to help you resolve the conflict with your parents. This anger and resentment could affect your ability to cope and thrive.

Dear Sue: *Does having a foreskin make the penis more sensitive to stimulation?*

Sue says: The answer is yes, because the head (glans) of the penis is covered, and thus it is protected from the friction of underwear and is more sensitive. Males always want to know if females prefer males who are circumcised. It is not the foreskin that they are attracted to; it is the guy at the other end of the foreskin. Seriously, a woman's reaction to a foreskin really depends on what she is expecting to see, what she is used to and her past experiences. It is up to you to prove her right or wrong.

The prospect of being circumcised as an adult can be scary, as the following letter indicates:

Dear Sue: *My foreskin is so tight that I am unable to retract it back over the head of my penis. Whenever I have sex, the skin tears and there is some bleeding and pain. Do I have to have a circumcision?*

Sue says: Relax. Very few doctors do a full circumcision on adult males. Doing a dorsal slit is much simpler with a faster recovery time—the doctor freezes the foreskin, and with surgical scissors make a small cut at the end of the foreskin, cauterizes or ties off any blood vessels that are bleeding, and then you are fine. Well, you may want to apply the old bag of frozen peas to reduce the swelling, and you may not be too gung ho about jogging or sex for the next few days, but you will be fine. So do see your doctor. Ongoing breaks in the foreskin leave you vulnerable to infections, including HIV/AIDS.

COCK RINGS

Dear Sue: *My boyfriend and I were having sex and I noticed he never lost his erection. When I went down on him, I noticed this pinkish plastic ring around his penis. I nearly died. He told me he ordered it from the back of a skin magazine. Is it dangerous? He thinks it is great. If it's safe, I think so, too.*

Sue says: These are called penile constricting devices or, in simpler language, cock rings, and are available from novelty stores, head shops, and men's sex magazines. Yes, they work, and yes, they can be dangerous if they are left on for too long.

To use the ring, when a guy has a full erection, he hooks his two index fingers into the ring, expands it as much as possible and rolls it down to the base of his penis, and leaves it there. This constricting ring traps the blood in his penis, so he is able to maintain his erection as long as he wants.

We tell guys not to leave it on for more than twenty minutes—half an hour, maximum. While the ring is on, there is no circulation of fresh, oxygen-rich blood to the penis. Without oxygen, after a while, tissue in the penis starts to die. Not good.

Removing a cock ring can be uncomfortable. He must hook his fingers under the ring to expand it, at which point the erection goes away. As he rolls the ring off, it snags and pulls on his pubic hair. Not fun. Using lots of lube makes removal easier.

Generally, these rings are used by male strippers or older men who are unable to maintain an erection long enough for satisfactory sex.

CONDOMS

Over and over I emphasize the necessity of using condoms, and I am going to explain in detail how to use one properly. I recommend that you use such brand-name condoms as Lifestyles, Sheik, or Trojan. They are tested and reliable, and will not tear or slip off if used properly. Do not use the "natural" or "skin" condoms. Supposedly they do not reduce sensation, but they are porous, so viruses or sperm can pass through them.

When you buy condoms, you must check the expiration date. Do not store condoms in your wallet or in the glove compartment of your car, because they deteriorate when they are old or are exposed to heat, cold, or light. Take a fresh package when you go out for a hot evening.

To use a condom, first open the package gently so that you do not tear the condom. Place it with the ring rolled up over the head of the penis and gently roll the condom right down to the base of the penis. Leave a little slack at the tip of the condom, gently squeezing the tip to expel the air. This leaves a space for your ejaculate to be stored, so the condom will not break.

Now, after sex, before you withdraw the penis from the vagina, hold on to the condom so it does not slip off and spill the ejaculate, which would leave your partner unprotected against infection and unplanned pregnancy. Do not use a condom twice.

There are a few things about condoms that are not generally known, so don't skip the next letters.

Dear Sue: *Last week I was having sex with a new guy in my life, and the condom slipped off. I flipped out. What should I do?*

Sue says: Well, at this point there is nothing you can do, but you could have immediately placed one applicator full of contraceptive foam into your vagina. That contains spermicide and germicide, which would have helped protect you. To protect himself, he could have urinated immediately when he got to a bathroom, and washed his genitals with soap and water. If either of you develops signs and symptoms of any sexually transmitted diseases, go to your family doctor or STD clinic immediately and don't have any sex until it is diagnosed, treated, and cured.

Dear Sue: *Halfway through sex, my genitals get sore, raw, red, and irritated. Peeing is painful. My doctor says I'm clear of* *infections. What could it be? It never happened with my last boyfriend.*

Sue says: This could be an infection that did not show up with testing. Go without sexual intercourse for a couple of weeks to allow your genitals to heal, which won't happen overnight. Then use a condom every time you have sex for about three months. If all is well at that point and you are in a stable, loving, and committed relationship, try sex without a condom and see if you have the same inflammation. If you do, try a different brand of condom.

If your genitals get sore again, there is a possibility that you are allergic to your partner's ejaculate. In that case you must continue to use condoms. If the time comes when you want to get pregnant, you will have to figure out exactly when you are ovulating and have unprotected sex at that time. Most times, though, these reactions resolve themselves—they flare up periodically and then subside.

Something else we must be aware of is that some people are allergic to latex. Try washing a new condom with soap and cool water to remove latex particles, and then apply a lubricant and roll up again for use. You could also use the new female condom, which is made of polyurethane, but they are expensive (see the question on the next page).

You may want to purchase lubricated condoms, but many HIV/AIDS services recommend that you not use condoms lubricated with the spermicide Nonoxynol 9. Unfortunately, it can be very irritating to the sensitive mucous membranes of genitals and leave them raw, red, sore, and vulnerable to infections, including AIDS. Lubricated condoms are great, but if you experience an allergic reaction, avoid those lubricated with spermicide/germicide.

Dear Sue: *How does the female condom differ from latex male condoms?*

Sue says: Yes, the condom for women is now available in North America. It is like a Baggie and it is not stretchy latex like the condoms we are used to. It has two flexible rings. One goes inside at the top to fit around the cervix. The other ring, located at the open end, prevents the condom from riding up into your vagina and keeps the condom open, outside the vaginal opening. If one partner has an infection, the female condom protects the other partner's genitals from contact with bacteria or virus (unlike the male condom, which offers less protection for women's genitals than for men's).

The female condom is 40 percent stronger than latex condoms, and protects against all sexually transmitted diseases. It looks weird, but is more comfortable than the male condom, and it transmits body heat so it feels more natural. Another plus: it can be inserted hours before sexual activity.

Unfortunately the female condom is expensive, at fifteen dollars for three, and it is one more method for females, so it lets men off the hook. However, it is the only type of condom that protects the female's genitals as well as the male's. Because of HIV/AIDS and other infections, women must be adamant about protection, whether their partners like it or not. We are responsible for our own Safer Sex. Then we never have to worry when he says, "That? Oh, that's just a blister."

CONTRACEPTION ADVANCES

Dear Sue: *My doctor prescribed tetracycline for me. Will the Pill still be effective?*

Sue says: Yes. The most recent research says that the Pill will continue to be effective as a contraceptive even if you are on tetracycline. However, there are some medications that seem to reduce the effectiveness of the Pill, so if you are using any of the following drugs, do use backup methods of birth control such as condoms and foam: barbiturates (sedatives), some sulfa drugs, some anti-inflammatory drugs, Dilantin (for epilepsy), and drugs to reduce blood pressure. Antacids may reduce the absorption of the medication in the Pill. If you require insulin, check with your doctor.

If you are on the birth-control pill, ask your pharmacist if the medication in any new prescription would reduce its effectiveness. Don't be shy, be sure.

Dear Sue: *I heard a short item on the radio that said they were researching a new male contraceptive, which is not yet available.*

Sue says: There are two or three methods of contraception currently being researched, but to date, the negative side effects make them impractical. Don't hold your breath for a long-term male method of birth control other than vasectomy

Dear Sue: *I can't take the Pill and my doctor was telling me about a new intrauterine device. I have two children and don't want any more right now.*

Sue says: The new intrauterine device (IUD), called Mirena, releases a small but constant amount of hormone that causes a thickening of the cervical mucus, preventing the passage of sperm into the uterus; in some women it stops ovulation. In the beginning, your periods may be heavier, but they become lighter after a few months. The IUD is effective for up to five years, but should you decide to have another baby, fertility returns after six months.

The doctor would insert Mirena during your normal menstrual period. Do have a routine pelvic exam, Pap smear, and tests for sexually transmitted diseases.

Dear Sue: *Our doctor recommended a birth-control injection for my eighteen-year-old daughter. Is it safe? She is a typical teen and might forget to take the Pill regularly.*

Sue says: Yes, Depo Provera is an effective contraceptive for folks who are negligent pill takers. Depo is a progesterone-only drug that is injected into her upper arm or "tush" every three months.

With continued use, your daughter's menstrual period will probably decrease, and after a year of use she will probably not have monthly periods. There may be some negative side effects, especially in the beginning; she may gain weight, suffer from headache, bloating, or depression. There is some concern that the shot may prevent calcium from being deposited in her long bones, at a time of her life when she should be storing calcium. Ask your doctor about this. Depo Provera averages out to about the same cost as the birth-control pill.

Dear Sue: *I heard that the Today sponge is now back. Is it true?*

Sue says: Yes, it is available in drugstores again. The sponge is a doughnut-shaped ring impregnated with the spermicide Nonoxynol 9. You wet the sponge, work up a lather, and insert it into your vagina, as high up as possible. There it traps, blocks, and kills sperm. You can remove it the next day by simply hooking your finger under the tape and sliding it out. Be aware that some people may develop an allergic reaction to Nonoxynol 9.

Dear Sue: *In* Time *magazine (November 19, 2001) I read about Nuvaring, a thin, flexible plastic ring that you insert into your vagina and leave there for twenty-one days. You then remove it, have a period, and insert another ring. They said it was comfortable and would not interfere with sex. The article said it would be available mid-2002. Is it available yet?*

Sue says: Yes, it is available. Do contact your doctor.

Dear Sue: *My girlfriend is on the birth-control pill, but she does not go off the Pill to have a period. She just keeps on taking the pill for three months, then she goes off for a week. Is this safe?*

Sue says: If she is on the correct birth-control pill, it is safe and effective. She should be on a monophasic prescription, twenty-one pills that contain the same strength of estrogen and progesterone for twenty-one days. When she has finished one package of twenty-one, she starts a new package the next day. She will not have a period, and she can do this for three months. Then she goes off the pills for seven days, has a period, and starts again for three months. Researchers say this is fine. They are working on new pills called Seasonale that you take nonstop for three months; then you go off for seven days and start again.

If she is on packages that contain twenty-eight pills, the last seven pills are sugar pills and must be discarded or she will have a period.

But, and this is important, if a woman is on triphasic birth-control pills, she can't do this. The hormones in the pills are different strengths depending on when in the cycle they're taken, and she could get pregnant. So before she tries this routine, she should see her doctor, Planned Parenthood, or a sexual health clinic.

Monophasic pills include: Ortho-Cept, Cyclen, Alesse, Demulin 30, Minovral, Loestrin, Marvelon, Brevicon, and Diane 35. Triphasic pills include: Tri-Clyclen, Triphasil, Ortho 10/11 or Ortho 7/7/7, and Triquilar, or Synphasic.

Again, do see a doctor or clinic before you embark on this program.

CYSTS, OVARIAN

Dear Sue: *I was having pain in my abdomen, which was worse at certain times of the month, and sex was agony most of the time. Occasionally, it would be just fine. My doctor says I have ovarian cysts. What are they?*

Sue says: The ovaries are small organs (about the size of an almond) located at the far end of the fallopian tubes, which are attached to the top of the uterus. Got the picture? Ovaries are glands that produce the essential female hormones estrogen and progesterone, which control the menstrual cycle and trigger the release of an ovum (egg) once a month. Ovaries also produce very small amounts of male sex hormones, or androgen.

Now this may surprise you, but male hormone makes women androgynous; that is, it gives them that wonderful combination of femaleness with a twist of the masculine component. And men produce small amounts of the female sex hormones, which make them capable of being gentle and tender. Don't fight these various components of your person-ality; they make you unique. But I digress . . .

Ovaries do not produce hormones until puberty. Then they function on a fairly regular cycle until females go into menopause, at about age fifty. About 3 percent of women in their reproductive years develop cysts on their ovaries, generally as a result of excess androgen production. These cysts occasionally flare up, can become as large as a grape-fruit, and then may recede until another time. Signs and symptoms include irregular and/or heavy menstrual periods, periodic low-back pain, infertility, discomfort or pain during intercourse, perhaps excess hair on the face, arms, and up-per chest, and sometimes acne that won't respond to treat-ment.

Your doctor will confirm the diagnosis by blood hormone profiles and ultrasound to locate the size and number of cysts.

After he has given you a diagnosis, your doctor may pre-scribe birth-control pills or progesterone-only pills, a drug to counteract androgen, or, as a last resort, surgery to remove the cysts.

You can keep an accurate record of the pain cycles of your menstruation. If sex is agony, try a different position, perhaps the knee-chest position (good old doggie-style sex). In this position, the uterus falls forward into your abdominal cavity, which means the penis will not bang into the cervix and push the uterus up, tugging on your ovaries to produce pain. Or you may try the woman-on-top position so that you can control the depth of thrusting and avoid the pain. Be innovative.

If sex is just unbearable, don't have intercourse. Fool around, do everything else like mutual masturbation (heavy-duty petting) or oral-genital sex, all of which are very pleasurable, satisfying, and will likely not provoke the pain.

Let me reassure you, ovarian cysts are not precancerous, but you should have regular annual checkups. It may be small comfort, but ovarian cysts usually settle down with the onset of menopause.

[d]

DEPRESSION

Depression appears to be the major distress of our era. Approximately 20 percent of Canadians experience severe, debilitating depression at least once during their lifetime, usually around midlife (although it can affect people of any age, including children and the elderly). About the same number of males as females suffer depression, although women are more likely to admit to the problem and seek professional help. According to some studies, people who are married or have a partner seem to suffer depression less frequently than those who are single, widowed, or divorced.

This letter clearly shows the "Five *D*s" of depression—defeated, defective, deserted, deprived, and diminished capacity.

Dear Sue: *I am having real difficulty coping with my wife because she is so sad and gloomy all the time. She does not sleep* *at night and she sits and stares at the wall like a zombie all day, no matter what I do to try to cheer her up. She drags me down with her, so I often work late because I get so tired trying to scrape her up out of the pits. She cries and blames herself for everything, gets confused, and will not go out with our family or friends. She just "vegges out" here alone.*

Sue says: I can almost feel you going down for the count, and am extremely concerned about many aspects of your letter. It sounds as though you are trying to meet all your wife's needs, alone.

In her depression, she has become totally dependent on you. You have moved into the rescuer mode, partially out of empathy, perhaps guilt, and a lot of fear that she will get worse or attempt suicide. You may feel this situation has no end. You may be worried about your ability to cope, and whether the relationship and marriage can survive.

I do hope that you can get good counseling for yourself as caregiver. For your own mental health, you must eat well, exercise, and get enough rest. You need some social outlets, so keep in contact with family and friends. This may mean enlisting their assistance to look after your wife while you take a break, go for a walk, have a swim, get a massage, or go to a movie. You have to look after yourself in order to be able to help your wife.

I am sure you have tried everything in your power to help her out of this depression, but here are a few suggestions for things to do together: relaxation tapes; a massage; a whirlpool or sauna; going to a mall; renting a light video to watch; or reading aloud from a funny book.

Could you encourage her family and friends to telephone her, not daily, but perhaps weekly, to chat with her? This will help convince her that others out there love her, and that she has not been forgotten. Do you have friendly neighbors with whom she feels comfortable who might invite her for coffee?

People who are depressed often benefit from dancing. Could the two of you take up folk dancing, square dancing, or ballroom?

Having specific tasks for which she is responsible every day might help her—washing the dishes, cleaning the kitty litter, watering the plants, buying a newspaper, peeling the potatoes for supper. Accomplishing something will help her to feel capable and competent; it will reduce her feelings of uselessness and dependency and raise her self-esteem. It is important that you praise and thank her if she does these tasks. If she wants to talk, do practice empathic listening, giving her encouragement, saying, for example, "I didn't know you felt that way. I am glad you told me."

Some strategies that have been recommended by certain therapists are not effective—crying, shouting, and banging pillows does not alleviate depression. Being alone can increase depression, and blaming others does not elevate one's mood. Surrendering to the blackness simply increases the depression.

This places a real burden on you. Do not try to go it alone. Arrange for daily respite care. There is absolutely no reason why you cannot tell your wife what you need: "I'd like to go for a bike ride," or "I need a hug," or "I need to know that you still love me, not as your caregiver, but as your partner." This, too, can make her feel needed and raise her self-esteem.

Even with this, I am sure there will be times when you want to say, "Get up off your ass and smarten up. There are other people in this world besides you." When these feelings come, get a journal and write them down. You do not need to feel guilty about having these thoughts; you did not ask for this burden and you may feel cheated. These are normal, healthy reactions and you should acknowledge them. I would hope you could find a good counselor to get you through this.

You need to know that depression is *not* self-induced. Telling her to pull herself out of it will not help. Most experts believe that depression may result when a number of stress factors and life experiences converge and trigger a breakdown. Sometimes it is biologically based; sometimes it is genetic. Research is being done to establish if there is a biochemical predisposition to clinical depression.

Bad moods and depression are contagious. Researchers say it takes only about twenty minutes of exposure to someone's depression to catch it. Some people are more sensitive to others' moods; these people are "receivers" and are inclined to feel guilty if they feel up when the other person is down.

It may be helpful for you to know that depression is often temporary. Perhaps you can reassure her that "this, too, will pass." Meanwhile, I hope you can find effective treatment, which will bring about improvement and recovery. Do ask your doctor about Prozac or other antidepressants. Although a few people experience negative side effects from it, for many clinically depressed people Prozac brings dramatic improvement, especially in conjunction with ongoing psychotherapy.

Hang in there, honey. You will get through this, and so will she.

DISABILITY

Each disability presents its own unique challenge to the individual to enjoy the best sex possible.

Dear Sue: *My eleven-year-old daughter has cerebral palsy, and it's time to talk sex with her. She is not verbal, but understands what we say. How do we do this?*

Sue says: In all probability, you have been giving her messages and information all along. Now you must be specific. Bliss Symbols International has developed symbols relating to sex and sexuality and these can be used with a Bliss board (a board of symbols depicting words or phrases). So you can talk to your daughter and read books together, and she will be able to ask questions as you go along. For more information about the Bliss board, contact your local cerebral palsy association.

I am impressed that you accept her sexuality, that she will have sexual urges, want to masturbate, and want an intimate, loving sexual relationship. She is a lucky lady to have you as a parent.

Perhaps you could help her teachers implement a good sex-education program in her school for other kids with disabilities who do not have sensitive parents such as you.

Carry on. You're on the right track. You may want to check out *The Ultimate Guide to Sex and Disability* by Miriam Kaufman, M.D., Cory Silverberg, and Fran Odette (San Francisco: Cleis Books, 2003).

Dear Sue: *In spite of the fact that my husband has arthritis, our sex life was good until he had a heart attack about six months ago. Since then, everything has been on hold.*

Sue says: Sounds as though you had learned to work around his arthritis. Being sure he was well rested, had a relaxing hot bath beforehand, took aspirin or other medication to ease his discomfort. This probably made sex possible and pleasurable. Of course, you would also have had to adapt your sexual moves to accommodate his arthritis.

You need to know you are both still sexual; that did not stop with his cardiac problems. By now he will be established on a regular exercise program. So if he can walk ten blocks or climb one flight of stairs without distress, he can safely have sex.

You may find it easier if you are on top (see the section on positions, page 00). Mutual stimulation, manual and oral-genital sex are less strenuous for people who tire easily. Try good old "69" with you on top.

Some medications may lower his sex drive and ability to attain or maintain an erection. Check that out with the doctor.

Many doctors and physiotherapists avoid talking about sex with their patients, and couples are reluctant to bring up the subject; they are afraid to talk to each other about their feelings, fears, concerns, and needs. They envisage their partner dying of a heart attack during sex. Very unlikely. Do discuss it, relax, and enjoy.

Two great books on this subject are *In Sickness and in Health: Sex, Love and Chronic Illness* by Lucille Carlton (New York: Delacourt, 1996), and *Enabling Romance: A Guide to Love, Sex and Relationships for the Disabled* by Ken Kroll and Erica Levy Klein (Toronto: No Limits, 2001).

DOCTOR/THERAPIST–CLIENT ABUSE

Dear Sue: *I had to go to my doctor because I was having pain during sex. He did a pelvic exam, but it was different. He was touching my genitals, inserting fingers into my vagina in a thrusting manner, and suddenly I realized he had taken his penis out. I was terrified and screamed for him to stop. He said he was trying to find out exactly where my pain was. His nurse came running in and I got the very strong feeling that this was not the first time this had happened as she tried to reassure me that I had imagined the exposed penis. The doctor insisted he was only trying to find out where my abdominal pain was.*

Sue, it has been three years and I haven't been to a doctor since. What should I do?

Sue says: The first thing I would recommend is that you find a nice female doctor whom you like and can trust. Before your exam, tell her what happened. After three years, you do need a medical checkup by a doctor who will be supportive and understanding and will refer you to a good counselor if you feel you need one.

I do not want to pressure you to lay assault charges on this doctor, but if you are feeling strong and positive, you can help protect other women from his medical malpractice by doing so. To do this, contact the American Medical Association and ask about the proper procedure to follow. Then write out your accusations and send the letter by registered mail to the association and to your lawyer, and find out if they will send a copy to the offending doctor.

Doctor-patient abuse is illegal, unethical, and immoral. Studies show that between 5 and 10 percent of patients, mostly females, suffer sexual abuse from doctors, psychologists, and therapists. There are some common patterns when doctors and therapists abuse their clients.

- The doctor/therapist usually has marital problems or is feeling sexually deprived. His client is generally about sixteen years younger than he is, and occasionally he believes he loves the client.
- Some doctors are convinced they are sexually involved with the patient because she is depressed or her self-confidence needs a boost, or some therapists may assert that they are acting as a surrogate in a teaching, hands-on capacity.

- Some therapists, primarily women, believe that if they give their client love he or she will be fine.
- Some therapists are needy and vulnerable. This puts the client who is seeking counseling in the role of helper/counselor for the counselor.
- The doctor/counselor may be convinced that the client was seductive, wanted sex, and that, being male, he succumbed to her charms.

The case may have to go to court. If it does, the doctor or therapist will be charged with sexual assault. The doctor's license will probably be lifted. He may be allowed to work in an administrative capacity but not as a practicing physician. You can also charge him with assault and battery in a civil lawsuit for monetary compensation.

It is well worth the effort to find a good doctor whom you like and trust. If you have repressed any anger over the experience and have become depressed as a result, there are new medications that can be very helpful for depression. And do find a counselor to work with. If you are ready, you can move from victim to survivor to winner.

[e]

ECTOPIC PREGNANCY

Dear Sue: *I had a tubal pregnancy a year ago and I nearly died. Now I am scared of trying to get pregnant again. What are my chances of having a full-term pregnancy and a normal baby?*

Sue says: The medical term for tubal pregnancy is "*ectopic pregnancy,*" and it may occur if one or both fallopian tubes are partially blocked by scar tissue from infection or the use of an IUD (an intrauterine contraceptive device) or bound up by adhesions, endometriosis, or ovarian cysts.

Normally, when you ovulate the egg is picked up by the open ends of the fallopian tubes and it rolls down the tube. If you have unprotected sex, sperm swim through the uterus and up into the tube. One sperm fertilizes the egg. That fertilized egg will continue to roll down the tube and plop into the uterine cavity where it becomes implanted. Then its cells multiply and differentiate to develop into a fetus.

However, if there is scar tissue from an infection (called pelvic inflammatory disease), which blocks the tube, when you ovulate, the egg rolls to the blockage but is stopped there. Now, sperm are a million times smaller than an egg, so they may pass through and impregnate the egg, but then this fertilized egg is stuck. Once fertilized, it starts to grow and develop in the tube. When the tube cannot stretch any farther, it ruptures, after about eight weeks.

This causes excruciating pain and bleeding into your abdomen, and you could go into shock and die if you do not get to a hospital quickly. In the operating room, you are given an anesthetic, and a doctor performs abdominal surgery to stop the bleeding, remove the embryo, and try to repair the fallopian tube with the hope that more scar tissue will not form to block the tube again. The tube may have to be removed if the damage is extensive.

Whether or not you will be able to conceive and sustain a healthy pregnancy depends on the present health of your fallopian tubes. The damaged one may have healed and remained open, and you still have the other tube; the doctor may want to check them to be certain they are patent (open). If not, you will be sterile, at least for now. You still have your ovaries, so you will continue to ovulate and menstruate.

If both tubes are blocked, there still may be a chance to repair them. Some gynecologists have developed a technique to surgically repair blocked tubes, but there are no guarantees. The fallopian tubes are only as thick as the lead of a pencil. Cutting out the damaged section, suturing the two ends together, and keeping an opening without more scar tissue is extremely difficult.

If your doctor suspects an ectopic pregnancy, or if you have a history of tubal pregnancies, as soon as you think you might be pregnant, your doctor will monitor you every week by transvaginal ultrasound. As soon as an ectopic pregnancy is diagnosed, the embryo will be surgically removed. This will prevent the tubal damage and hemorrhaging that would ensue if the tube ruptures.

Extensive research is being done with a drug that would cause a tubal pregnancy to be aborted before it caused complications.

Do read on because if all else fails, there is always in vitro fertilization.

ENDOMETRIOSIS

Dear Sue: My life sucks. I am a thirty-two-year-old woman. I have a great boyfriend whom I adore, but I spend about half my life in agony. I am doubled over about midcycle for ten days before menstruation starts and a few days after. The rest of the time, I'm scared sex will hurt. My doctor is going to start testing for endometriosis. What am I in for? Do they have any effective treatment?

Sue says: It's small comfort, but at least your doctor isn't telling you, "It's all in your head." When you said that sex was painful, you did not say if the pain occurred at a certain point in your cycle or if it is constant. If there are times when you are pain-free or are able to manage the pain, then enjoy glorious, uproarious sex. Other times, perhaps you could stimulate him. He can also be responsible for his own sexual pleasure when you are just not into it. This is workable.

Now to get to the tough stuff. We don't know why endometriosis is becoming more common, but it can be debilitating, hard to diagnose, and even harder to treat. There is some evidence that endometriosis is hereditary. It is caused by tissue from the lining of the uterus being displaced through the fallopian tubes into the abdominal cavity. This tissue may adhere to your bowel, uterus, and fallopian tubes, and may migrate to other parts of your abdomen. When the female hormones that trigger ovulation and menstruation are released, this displaced tissue reacts, causing abdominal pain and even bleeding into the abdomen. For some women it is negligible, for others, excruciating. Some women also experience pain during bowel movements, and others have pain in their lower back or legs.

There appears to be a connection between chronic yeast infections and endometriosis. If you have any signs of a yeast infection, get it treated promptly. (For symptoms of yeast infections, see page 287.)

To diagnose endometriosis, your doctor will do a careful pelvic examination to locate tender areas, nodules, or ovarian cysts. An ultrasound will be done next to help locate stray tissue and cysts.

An ultrasound is safe and painless, but it can be uncomfortable because you have to drink liters of water to fill your bladder until after the ultrasound. You feel as though you are going to explode! Next, your abdomen is well lubricated and a small handheld instrument, traced over your abdomen like a computer mouse over a mouse pad, bounces sound waves off your internal organs. These sound waves are transmitted to a monitor or screen, producing a flat image of your insides. If endometrial cysts are present, they should show up on the monitor.

If an ultrasound shows endometrial tissue, the doctor will do a laparoscopy (while you are under general anesthetic) so he or she can locate exactly where the endometrial tissue is located in your abdomen.

A few surgeons are using a laparoscope to slowly and carefully remove the abnormal tissue. It can be done by electrocautery or laser, but that causes scar tissue, which may result in adhesions.

Unfortunately, when you have a confirmed diagnosis, there is no cure—though there are several treatments. Even with the best treatment, endometriosis may recur. Treatment involves trial and error, and is tricky. Depending on the frequency and severity of your pain, antiprostaglandin medication may be prescribed, which should help. You may be given low-dose birth-control pills, but these can have side effects, such as tender breasts and no periods. Keep your doctor informed.

Danazol is a powerful drug that stops ovulation and menstruation, and is sometimes used to treat endometriosis. The theory behind this treatment is, if you eliminate the hormones, you eliminate the extra-uterine tissue reaction, and therefore the pain. This works for many women, but there are a few problems. You can only take the medication for eight or nine months, and cysts may return after you go off the drug. Danazol is a derivative of the male hormone testosterone, so it may have masculinizing effects. Your breasts may shrink, you may develop facial hair and/or acne, your voice may become lower, and you may gain weight. These changes can be permanent. But Danazol is very effective for many women and is an alternative to surgery.

Pregnancy has the same effect as Danazol, so if you want to have a baby someday, now might be a good time, especially since the cysts might get worse, making it more difficult to get pregnant. If you are having difficulty getting pregnant because of endometriosis, a six-week course of Danazol may be effective. The success rate is between 40 and 50 percent.

There is a new treatment by the trade name of Synarel that produces a pseudo menopause. It is very expensive and also has some negative side effects, including hot flashes, vaginal dryness, headaches, depression, mood swings, low sex drive, and decreased bone density, which can lead to osteoporosis. We do not know the long-term side effects on fertility, so this drug should be used only once for no longer than six months. Researchers have only now discovered that the intrauterine device Mirena reduces the number and severity of endometriosis attacks.

If your endometriosis is very serious and does not respond to any therapy, the doctor might suggest a hysterectomy to remove your uterus and ovaries. Before you go that route, you might consider doing some serious research and experimenting with alternative treatments. Check out naturopathic and homeopathic treatments, acupuncture, visualization, and relaxation. You may find some combination that works for you. Some women have found that a macrobiotic diet is effective.

I would love to be able to offer you a cure on a platter, but it is just not there. By the slow process of elimination, you will have to find what works for you. At least it does not go on forever. Endometriosis disappears with menopause— small consolation when you are thirty-two and in love. But I have a few more suggestions for getting help.

The Endometriosis Association provides information and support for women who suffer from endometriosis. Contact them at 8585 N. Seventy-sixth Place, Milwaukee, WI 53223; phone 414-355-2200; fax 414-355-6065; www.endometriosisassn.org. An excellent book on the subject is *The Endometriosis Source-*

book by Mary Lou Ballweg and the Endometriosis Association (New York: McGraw-Hill, 1995). *Gynecological Health* by M. Sara Rosenthal (New York: McGraw-Hill, 2003), 4th ed., is another helpful resource.

EROTICA AND PORNOGRAPHY

Say the word "pornography" and watch most women react, some with feelings ranging from dismay to revulsion. They have this knee-jerk reaction not because they are prudish, nor because of feminist indoctrination. It appears to be a spontaneous gut response to visual depictions of sexual activity that they consider unrealistic, abnormal, exploitive of women, and, some would say, disgusting. Many males see pornography as harmless, fun, and titillating.

This letter gives us an idea of the way women feel.

Dear Sue: I was at my boyfriend's place and I found a pile of Playboy *magazines. I glanced at a few, and although they weren't my cuppa tea, they appeared harmless, so I didn't get all upset. Later, he plugged in a porn video and we started watching. Sue, it was filth, abusive and violent. He thought it was great. I left. He apologized the next day, said he'd never do it again, and I accepted that—till last week when I found another skin magazine by his bed. Now don't get me wrong, he is a really great guy and I love sex with him, but this scares me and it also turns me off. What's to do?*

Sue says: Sounds as though you are feeling deceived and disappointed. He lied, so can you trust him again? You thought your sex life was great, so why does he have this compulsion to watch what you see as repulsive, abnormal sex? You may feel that your body will never compare to "Betsy Big Boobs" and wonder if that's what he wants in a partner. Is he addicted to the stuff? In the future, is he going to want to act out some of the scenes in these videos? Could it escalate to kiddie porn or snuff videos? These questions are very threatening for most women.

Don't get me wrong, most females enjoy erotica, which is softer, gentle, romantic, loving, and sexy. This explains the popularity of Harlequin romances. There are also erotic videos available, which most females enjoy. But pornography often depicts forceful sex where the female, unwilling in the beginning, becomes awed by the hero's huge "member." After much pushing and shoving, she loves it. This is not reality.

So what's a lady to do? Well, she really has to be very, very clear about how she feels, why she is reacting this way, why it makes her uncomfortable, and what she is afraid of. Then, without ranting and raving, she has to explain this to her boyfriend, talk about fear, feeling used, vulnerable, inadequate, and turned off. He needs to understand that she is going to need time to build up the trust level again. And she needs to make it very clear that she feels very strongly about this and that if it continues, she will break up with him.

True, some couples can watch porn videos together, find them very stimulating, and use them for arousal, but they are not generally hard-core porn films, so it's not a problem.

I must confess, I have a great concern about kids watching porn in videos or on the Internet. Many families lock off the pornography on the Internet, but kids may have friends who watch their parents' porn videos or watch it on the Internet. All they have to do is go to a friends' house to watch it. Teens are getting much of their sex education from porn videos, which do not depict sex in a loving, caring, committed relationship.

Another letter, a little unusual, but interesting:

Dear Sue: *My boyfriend does not live in my city, and we only see each other once a month. What do you think about us making a video of us having sex that he could have when I am not there?*

Sue says: Well, this puts a whole new twist on the home-movie industry. You won't be showing this along with the video of Junior's first birthday party. And therein lies the problem. What if this relationship breaks up? Who gets the video? If you don't get it, perhaps it will be shown at a stag night and someday you will be recognized in the grocery store as "Miss Hot-to-Trot." In reality, your partner could sell it. Your partner could give it to your new husband as a wedding gift. If you do stay together as a couple, how are you going to feel thirty years from now if you have stretch marks and cellulite from here to there, and your partner, with a delicious sense of humor, decides to review the old passion play? What if your kids get hold of it: "Mommy, what are you and Daddy doing?" And if they are teens when they find it: "Mom, how come you won't let me do that?" Do consider the endless possibilities, and if you are really convinced that this is a great idea, then it's up to you.

One woman told me she took pictures of herself in a seductive pose, put one in with her partner's lunch pail. At noon, he was with the guys, and opened his lunch to find more than a bologna sandwich. Cheesecake! The other guys really enjoyed a good laugh, and he was embarrassed.

So it is up to you, but a safe rule of thumb is, never put on paper or film what you would not want to appear on the front page of the *National Enquirer*.

EXPECTATIONS

Dear Sue: I sometimes watch soap operas, and it seems that all the situations revolve around sex. Is sex all that important in our lives?

Sue says: When we are young, many of us have totally unrealistic expectations of what sex will be like. As teens, we do not know much about sex, only what we can glean from our friends; from sex education in school, which focuses on body parts but not "what goes where, when, why, and how"; from afternoon soaps that portray red-hot lust, or a lecture from Mom that started out with "now you are a woman," or for guys, "just don't get her pregnant" from Dad.

At a very early age, you discovered that it felt good to play with yourself, and you may have learned that your parents reacted strongly if they caught you at it. You learned that "fuck" was a no-no word, but you did not know what it meant. "Shit" was also a no-no word, but you knew what that meant.

You learned that love and sex go together, but Mommy and Daddy, who are supposed to be in love, don't do it. What's wrong with this picture? If you ever caught your parents "doing it," you did not talk about it. In fact, not talking about it seemed to be the rule.

You felt "youthfully disadvantaged" if, as a guy, you had these embarrassing, spontaneous erections that other guys called "popping a boner," but yours happened almost continuously. You went to sleep with one and you woke up with one—it just never went down. You decided you must be oversexed and a pervert.

If you are a female, you may have felt "pubescently challenged" when you had these restless feelings and got all "squishy" down there. You thought it was gross. You thought you were a nymphomaniac for life.

Then you heard that you were in your sexual prime, and soon it would all be downhill. And for guys, that seemed to be true. You still had erections, but not as often, nor as hard. Sometimes you would lose it before you began; other times you would blast off, out of control.

Females heard that they should come into their prime in their late twenties, and that scared them because if they were feeling this horny at eighteen, God help them when they were twenty-five. Here are some other common, unreal expectations:

- If you are in love, the passion will last forever.
- Your partner will know exactly how to turn you on.
- You will both have this cataclysmic simultaneous orgasm every time you have sex.
- You will never get pregnant accidentally, and when you want to get pregnant, it will happen immediately.
- Females are allowed to cry but not be sexy. Males are allowed to be sexy but are not allowed to cry.
- You will stay young, beautiful, and appealing for life.

Nobody tells you otherwise, but you are sexual for life. It does change and evolve, yes, and it does get better if you let it. That's what this book is all about.

It may not be easy. Growth is never painless. You have to be open to new ideas. You will have to drag out your old value system, that set of beliefs, some based on fact, some based on the need of your parents, society, and the church to control sexuality. You are going to have to examine what you learned in the light of new information and ask yourself,

"Why am I uncomfortable with that? Who told me that was wrong? Why did they think it was wrong? Is it really wrong? If not, am I going to let this attitude and value that is not really mine control my behavior for the rest of my life? If not, then what am I going to do about it?"

There are three components to personal growth: knowledge, information, and changing your behavior as a result of this new information. It is hard work and it can be really scary. If you have a partner, it is easier if you share your thoughts as they develop, and grow together. If you don't, your partner will notice a change and not understand it, feel threatened and cling to the security of the way things used to be (the good old days). Your partner may not follow your thought processes, may not agree with your conclusions, and that is okay, too, because at least he or she knows and understands your changes.

Partners have a choice: they can accept this new you and enjoy, or they can find they just cannot go along with you, and they can leave. That's why it is scary, but staying stuck is even scarier.

I try to remain value neutral. My role is to give you information and then you have to do the work. But I will push you, challenge you, and what you do with that is up to you.

[f]

FAKING ORGASM

Dear Sue: *How can a guy tell if his partner is faking orgasm? We've been together for three years and she says she "cums" but I'm not sure.*

Sue says: This is a tough one. Movies and TV show women apparently having these earth-shattering orgasms, so women who see these images think the way you should have an orgasm is to moan and groan, thrash, clutch, claw, and scream. They decide, "I can do that." Some women should be given an Academy Award for their performance of faking it. Truth is, there is really no sure way for you to be certain. Some orgasms really are this earth-shattering; many are mellower, more subtle, but still lovely.

One thing she can't fake is arousal. If she is lubricated, her genitals are wet, she is interested in sex, no fooling.

If she says she is happy, contented, and satisfied, you are going to have to take her word for it.

Somehow we have bought into the concept that women must have an orgasm every time they have sex, or they become cranky and frustrated—"instant bitches." But it does not work that way. Sometimes she has sex, and it feels good and she enjoys the touching, hugging, and holding, and she likes the feeling of togetherness. She is pleased that he is satiated, and although she did not have an orgasm, she is fine.

When a male is sexually aroused, he will probably have an erection; he will lubricate, and with stimulation, he will ejaculate and it feels good. He is satisfied by the ejaculation. Then every once in a while sex will be over-the-top spectacular, and that was orgasm for him. Men are smart enough to know it won't happen every time—if it does, it is amazing, and if not, sex is still satisfying and good. He's fine, too.

Females are the same. They do not need, nor do they expect, fireworks every time. So guys are going to have to trust their partner. If she says she is happy, believe her. Please do not ask, "Didja come?" She will let you know, "Wow, that was spectacular!" If it wasn't, one hopes she can be honest and say, "Well no, but it was wonderful, and you are terrific. I really enjoyed it and I feel great."

Take the pressure off yourself—you are not a flop as a lover if she does not go over the top every time. When you take the pressure off yourself, you take the pressure off her, too. No longer does she have to be theatrical; you can both relax and enjoy. There's more to sex than orgasm. If you don't accept that, you may find yourself with this problem . . .

Dear Sue: *I have never had an orgasm and I want one, but I have been faking it for years. How do I tell my partner?*

Sue says: What are your reasons for faking it? People do it for different reasons:

- To get it over with so you can go to sleep.
- Because his sexual-performance ego is a little wobbly, you decide to convince him he can move mountains.
- Perhaps you are trying to convince yourself that you really are having an orgasm.
- Perhaps you are worried that he will think you are frigid if you don't reach that climax.
- If you are having an outside affair, could you be trying to convince your partner he is the only one?

Can you reach orgasm by solitary masturbation? Because if you can, why do you want to tell your partner that you have been faking it? I am in favor of honesty, provided we do not use it as a weapon against our partner to make him feel like a lousy lover. Most women have their first orgasm all by themselves through solitary masturbation. If you know what brings you to orgasm, then you can very discreetly guide him to perform those things without putting him down.

If you have not been able to reach orgasm by any means, you may need to learn to masturbate to pleasure yourself. Then you can tell your partner you want to try your new moves.

An orgasm is not a gift you give to your partner; it is a gift you give yourself. However, I strongly suspect that any woman who claims she reaches orgasm every time is lying.

Dear Sue: *Can a guy fake orgasm?*

Sue says: Absolutely. Women do not have a monopoly on drama. He can make all the appropriate noises and be very convincing. If he did not use a condom, you might be aware the ejaculate was missing, but if he used a condom, then, really, you might not know he did not ejaculate or reach orgasm. A male who suffers from delayed ejaculation sometimes fakes it just to convince his partner that she is still sexy, and that she is a good lover.

Faking orgasm is not a great idea. You feel dishonest, and you may eventually avoid having sex because you are expected to put on a great show. A partner who suspects you have been faking it will be upset. It can jeopardize the honesty and trust in your relationship. Meanwhile it becomes a vicious cycle—she worries and becomes anxious, her arousal level goes down, reducing her chance of orgasm, which increases her anxiety and fear of being discovered, and on it goes. Honesty is the best policy.

FANTASY

What a boring, mundane existence we would have were it not for fantasy. Not only does it provide escape, it gives us sexual scenarios that are new, exciting, and different. Fantasies do not compete with sexual activity, nor do they interfere with it. Instead, they can influence and enhance sexual pleasure.

Most of the time, fantasies can add a whole new dimension if you are in a relationship. If the trust level is high, and you both share your fantasies, and you mutually agree to add some of them to your sexual repertoire, you can have great fun.

Let's say you have always thought it would be fun to have sex in a rocking chair. It's possible—just don't use that heirloom chair! Experiment with humor in another one—he sits, she straddles him, her legs over the chair's arms, and "if it's rocking, don't bother knocking."

You may have a fantasy that you just know your partner will definitely not go for, not out of prudishness, but just because it doesn't appeal. Your fantasy is your private property, to share or not to share. Enjoy it yourself.

Here are some interesting facts about fantasy:

- Men tend to daydream about real events, whereas women's daydreams are most often about imaginary situations. Female fantasies usually involve romantic situations, wooing, and courtship. Everybody fantasizes during masturbation.
- A fantasy may start out with one person in mind but generally that image changes to become vague and nebulous.
- During sex, most people fantasize about somebody else at times. This is normal, but unfortunately many people feel guilty, embarrassed, and ashamed. Some feel they are being unfaithful.
- In male sexual fantasies, he generally takes on a more active, dominant role, whereas in female sexual fantasies, she sees herself as more passive and as receptive and swept away by passion.
- A substantial number of both males and females fantasize they are being forced to have sex. A few may fantasize forcing somebody else to have sex against their will.
- Fortunately, most people who fantasize rape scenes are able to differentiate between fantasy and reality and do not attempt to turn their fantasy into reality.
- For most people, fantasizing does not increase the likelihood that they will act out their fantasies.

A couple of excellent books on fantasy are *Erotic Interludes: Tales Told by Women* (New York: Penguin, 1995), and *Pleasures: Women Write Erotica* (New York: Perennial, 1985) by Lonnie Barbach, Ph.D. These books provide fodder for some new and exciting sexual daydreams. You may realize that your old fantasies are dull, boring, and monotonous. Now you may explore and expand your repertoire of sexual fantasies. The most common concern about sexual fantasies is expressed in the next letter.

Dear Sue: *I am a straight twenty-seven-year-old male who occasionally imagines what it would be like to have sex with another guy. On the subway, I'll see a gay guy, great bod, nice tan, tight buns, bulge where a bulge should be, and I flip into this fantasy. Does this mean I am homosexual or bisexual?*

Sue says: Sounds like good fantasy material to me. Occasional same-sex fantasies are not a reliable indication of sexual preference. If they are your frequent favorites, if you also enjoy the company of women but are generally not turned on by women, and find yourself attracted to and seeking out specific males for companionship, and if this has been happening for some time, then your intuition may be accurate. But it is not something you have to decide by midnight tonight. Do not label yourself as homosexual till you are convinced you are correct.

There are times when you do have to be concerned about fantasies:

Dear Sue: *I really get turned on by fantasies of having sex with young kids. I get horny when I watch kids playing and I am afraid I might lose control.*

Sue says: This really scares me. First, you do not *lose* control, you *let go* of control. It is a nondecision decision. You unconsciously say to yourself, "I'm not going to fight this urge. It's bigger than I am and I am powerless." Wrong. At this point you have to get a grip on yourself. This is a fantasy and must remain a fantasy. You do not have the right to impose your fantasy on somebody else. What you are talking about is pedophilia. It is sexual abuse of a child and as such is a criminal offense. You must find a good therapist, a psychiatrist or psychologist, who can help you deal with these fantasies so that you do not act them out.

FETAL ALCOHOL SYNDROME

Dear Sue: *What is fetal alcohol syndrome? We have an opportunity to adopt a child who has been diagnosed as having it.*

Sue says: Fetal alcohol syndrome, or FAS, is a group of symptoms that appears in babies born to mothers who drank alcohol heavily during pregnancy. The babies typically have a small head, sloping forehead, with distinctive eyes and mouth. They suffer from neurological impairment and generally have a learning disability. Parenting FAS children can be difficult because of their inability to learn from experience, their short attention span, and lack of concentration. They are also generally hyperactive.

On the other hand, these children are very loving and capable of learning if they attend special educational facilities. It takes a very special family to give these kids the love and attention they need.

I am often asked, "How much can you drink during pregnancy?" There is no known safe amount of alcohol. In a study at the University of Western Ontario, there was evidence that one drink (one beer, one glass of wine, or one shot of liquor) reduced the fetal circulation to the brain by 30 percent. So, to be safe and sure, don't drink at all.

If you are considering adopting an FAS child, why not make arrangements to be a child's foster parents for six months to get some idea about whether you would be interested in an adoption? To you, I'd say, "God bless."

FETISH

I get many letters and calls from folks who find they become sexually aroused by specific objects or body parts not generally considered erotic.

A person has a fetish when he or she is unable to be sexually satisfied without that particular object being present, even with other stimulation.

It is difficult to draw the line as to what is normal and what is abnormal. Many males are aroused by breasts; some are "leg men." Many women are aroused by "tight buns." These are not considered abnormal, whereas someone who is turned on only by feet, or women who get turned on only by guys wearing leather, may be diagnosed as having a fetish.

Dear Sue: *I love women's feet. On the subway, I sometimes see a female with tanned feet and painted toenails wearing sandals and I want to kiss her feet, suck her toes, stroke her instep, and I have to get off the train. When I am with my girlfriend, I spend more time loving her feet than the rest of her. I stroke my genitals with her foot. Do I have a problem?*

Sue says: If you or your partner sees it as a problem, then it is a problem. A foot fetish is harmless; if it is acceptable to your partner and you can incorporate that stimulation into your foreplay-arousal pattern, then no problem. But if your partner starts to feel like a nonentity because you are more devoted to her foot than you are to her, your relationship may start to disintegrate. Basically, a fetish becomes a problem when it is the only way you can become aroused, or if you resort to manipulation, coercion, forced threats or exploitation of a partner to get what you want.

Besides feet, there are a wide variety of fetishes: hair, high-heeled shoes, or thigh-high boots, silky lingerie, leathers, and furs.

Other behaviors that could also be considered a fetish are diapering, light spanking, or scratching. In these activities the person becomes aroused by degradation (being scolded or punished for messing his or her diaper).

At present, there is no definitive explanation for why a person develops any particular fetish. Most fetishes seem to originate in early childhood from a particular event that resulted in pleasurable sexual stimulation. As the person matured, that object or behavior was incorporated into foreplay, eventually escalating into a full-blown fetish.

If your fetish interferes with the intimacy of your loving relationship, then it is advisable to seek therapy. In all probability, a psychologist or psychiatrist is the best-qualified person to provide effective counseling. A fetish is not a mental illness; it is classed as a perversion, not a deviancy.

You need to have good communication with your partner. If she starts to feel anger or resentment or is turned off by your attention to her feet, go for counseling for yourself in the beginning, and then for relationship counseling later on.

There's a great book that covers uncommon sexual practices, including fetishes. *The Sexually Unusual: A Guide to Understanding and Helping* by Dennis M. Dailey (New York:

Haworth Press, 1989) also covers sadomasochism, transvestism, transsexualism, exhibitionism/voyeurism, phone sex, and pedophilia. It is unlikely this book will be in your local bookstore, so you may have to order it, but it is well worth the wait.

FIBROIDS

Dear Sue: I am a healthy thirty-six-year-old married woman with three kids, and over the past six months I have been having periods from hell. They last two weeks, and I flood, literally. I am confined to bed with an ice bag, and if I do get up to go to the bathroom, the blood just gushes out with big clots. The doctor says I have fibroids. He says they are not cancerous but that they will probably not go away with menopause, and there is really nothing to do but remove them. Is this true?

Sue says: This is a classic history of fibroids. They are dense, heavy growths of fibrous tissue, tumors that develop on the top of the uterus, which can cause heavy bleeding, severe cramps, low-back pain, interfere with ovulation, and make pregnancy risky. We don't know what triggers fibroids, and at this point in time the best cure is surgery. A new surgery, called hysteroscopic myomectomy, uses electrical current to cut the fibroids off the uterine wall. The tumors are then removed through the cervix. You will not be able to carry a pregnancy after this surgery.

Uterine fibroid embolization is another new procedure, done under fluoroscopy. The doctor inserts a plastic catheter into the blood vessels that feed the tumor. They then release tiny plastic particles, blocking the blood vessels. The fibroids shrink by an average of 40 to 50 percent within one year.

There are concerns that after this procedure larger fibroids will develop a new blood supply and come back.

When your doctor discussed surgery, did he discuss the possibility of a hysterectomy if the fibroid was too large or too embedded in the uterus?

At this point, you are probably ready to flush the whole works down the toilet, but before you decide, read the section on page 144 on hysterectomy. Knowing that fibroids shrink after menopause may affect your decision.

FLIRTING

Interesting. If a female does it, it's called flirting and is regarded as a harmless pastime; whereas if a guy does it, he is on the prowl, on the make, and females feel he is "coming on to them." Because of the fear of being accused of sexual harassment, many males and females are reluctant to flirt.

Actually, flirting is wonderful if it is done in appropriate circumstances. You are at a party, dancing up a storm, and looking good. Then it would be fine to flirt. It wouldn't mean you were out to make a sexual conquest or asking to be raped.

To be a flirt, you need to know you are attractive, fun, and spontaneous, that you have some spark, like attention, and have the chutzpah to carry it off. Some people never do have it, but most will acquire it by their late teens, twenties, or early thirties. It never dies. Flashes of flirtatiousness will appear when the situation warrants it.

As adults, some women never give themselves permission to flirt when it is appropriate and safe, to do a "bump-and-grind" dance to attract her partner. The same goes for men; they may not dare make like Tarzan in a loincloth. All this is fun and can melt the ice or break the monotony of long-term love.

Researchers have found that there are fifty-two different nonverbal acts both males and females engage in during the "dance of attraction." It takes about fifteen seconds to grab the other's attention. Females use definite head movements, look coy, toss their hair, thrust their pelvis slightly forward, smile receptively, gaze attentively, or touch lightly. These all indicate interest.

Males seek out a woman, approach her, talk to her with intensity while standing close to her, and then back off a bit to recoup, then move closer again. They look at her with adoration, are solicitous, and use a very safe subtle touch—brushing her sleeve. If the touch is reciprocated, then that is interpreted as a go-ahead and he continues making advances until she rebuffs him or he decides that she is not interesting to him.

Some flirtatious behavior by males or females can present problems:

Dear Sue: *We are engaged, but you would never know it by the way my girlfriend struts her stuff with all my friends. She gets quite indignant if they take her up on her offer. Then she expects me to get her out of her mess.*

Sue says: There is a very fine line between flirting and cock teasing. Flirting is attention-getting behavior, a way of getting the four big As we all need: attention, approval, acceptance, and appreciation. It makes recipients feel good and strokes their egos. This takes skill and you have to know when to put the brakes on. Your partner has to know you and trust that you know what you are doing and are in control. Problems arise if either of you has been drinking or doing drugs. Then the line of discretion gets blurred and interpretation is up for grabs.

In our society, many people seem to be naturally flirtatious. Many little girls flirt with their fathers, with their uncles, flipping their curls and flaring their party dress, and we think it is cute. As soon as a girl enters puberty, it is no longer cute; it is seen as manipulative and is discouraged.

Occasionally, the flirtatious behavior is not discouraged and some females continue, not realizing it is inappropriate, might be misinterpreted, and could be downright risky.

So now we need to try and assess why your fiancée is into heavy-duty flirting. She may:

- Be worried that you do not find her attractive.
- Need more of the four big As.
- Be getting even with you for something you have done.
- Want to break the engagement or end the relationship.

People flirt to make their partner jealous, and to prove they are still attractive to others. This is a no-win situation because your partner may see you as cheap and foolish, turn against the person you are flirting with, blow their cool and get into a brawl, or walk away and never look back. Any which way, you lose.

Accusing your girlfriend of being a slut and expressing your anger by going home without her, avoiding parties and socializing, or breaking up is not the answer. Obviously you care for this lady. Let her know how her behavior makes you feel—tell her it embarrasses you, makes you uncomfortable with your friends, and that she does not need to prove how attractive she is. It's okay to be cute and coy, but you would feel better if she could moderate her behavior.

Generally, males are less subtle flirts, and most females sense what they are up to and will play along, but it is a game. Unfortunately, there are needy people who fall, hook, line, and sinker, for a smooth-talking man. They are vulnerable because, at best, they are going to get hurt; at worst, they are easy targets for sexual assault.

FORGIVENESS

Dear Sue: My husband had an affair for two years with his secretary. Everybody knew but me. I was devastated, but we have three kids and I do not want to leave. He says he is sorry, but I am unable to let it go. It is on my mind all the time and I am afraid it will do in our family life. Help!

Sue says: In all probability, you need to hear him ask for forgiveness, and he needs to hear you give forgiveness. But you will have to go deeper than words to rebuild lost trust, the love, and the intimacy. To do that, you need to look at what happened along the way.

When you started going out together, ground rules were established, unspoken expectations—you say you love me so you will protect me, not hurt me. You also agreed on a fundamental belief system. You believed that you could predict his behavior. "He just would not do that to me."

Now you feel you can no longer rely on him, and perhaps even worse, you feel you can no longer rely on yourself. Major problem: you chose this person, and you chose to believe in him. You wonder, "How could I have been so stupid? How could I have been so far off base?" You question your values, your faith, and your talents.

You were robbed. Every hope and dream you had for the

future has been shattered. You will not get over that loss to-morrow.

You feel as though you have no control over your life. That other person is calling the shots. And the person who was supposed to protect you is now the enemy. Now, whom do you trust? All old rules are up for grabs and you have to make new ones.

The unnerving part is that you probably still love and care for this person. He has hurt you and you are angry and filled with hate. You have lost so much that you are not willing to risk losing more.

I want to tell you, this is not hopeless. There are steps to help you move toward forgiveness. Get a journal and work your way through the following process. It's not fun, but it will help you move beyond being stuck in self-destructive ha-tred. Ready?

- List all the bottom-line rules of your relationship, rules that were broken. Include things like agree-ments on finances, "time together is sacred," hon-esty, and being faithful to each other. List everything you can think of.
- Who made those rules and when were they made, and were they ever spoken or were they tacit as-sumptions? Were they mutual or is it possible that your partner had different expectations?
- Are those rules realistic and reasonable? Be honest here. Are they still important to you or could you modify them?
- Now list the injuries that occurred when the rules were broken. You were deceived, the trust you placed in your partner was shattered. Now you don't

trust yourself or anybody else; you fear you look foolish with your friends and family.

- Is this injury permanent? How long will it take to heal?

You will realize that you have no control over what happened, but you do have control over the way you behave in response to his infidelity, so you are not totally powerless.

You will conclude that your life and your relationship have completely changed; the rules went out the window, so you have to make new ones. Whom can you trust and on what basis? What is fair and just? What can you control in your life?

You can develop stronger relationships with old friends and family. Make new friends and develop new interests. This will help you in the process of regaining power. If you can do this, you will be well on your way, but you are not done yet.

Calmly and rationally talk to the person about your injuries and honestly share what happened and how you are feeling.

- Admit that you were devastated, that you felt betrayed, powerless, and alone. Talk about your anger and fear, not accusing your partner, but telling him, "This is how it is for me right now."
- Admit that you are shattered. Don't pretend that nothing has happened. It has, and you are suffering. And the wound is not going to heal quickly. You are scarred for life; it will always be part of you, and that is not all bad.
- Acknowledge that it hurts less as time goes on.
- Move on to identify why he was unfaithful. Try to find a reason. Called blaming, this process is not the same as seeking revenge. You can blame his parents, his past, but mostly him. He had a choice to make,

and you accept that your behavior had some bearing on his decision to have an affair.

Now you are ready to forgive, and that too is a process. The damage is done, and now you must try to repair your relationship.

You need to tell him firmly that what he did was wrong. His behavior was unacceptable. He deserves punishment, not revenge. He may apologize and say he is sorry. He may even ask for forgiveness. You have done all the groundwork, so you will likely be able to forgive, but your relationship will have a different basis. Consider individual and/or couple counseling. An affair provides a chance to change a relationship for the better, or to end a bad one and get on with life.

You owe him nothing. He does not have power over you; you are responsible for yourself; you have a support system now, new friends, new interests, and new power. You will not forget completely and you will look back, but not with rancor. You will continue to grow and develop new dreams and expectations. You are now wiser and less vulnerable and needy. You are a winner because you refused to let the injury be terminal.

If you want more insight, do read *After the Affair* by Janis Abrahms Spring, Ph.D., with Michael Spring (New York: Perennial, 1997), *How Can I Forgive You?* by Janis Abrahms Spring, Ph.D., with Michael Spring (New York: HarperCollins, 2004), or *Having Love Affairs* by Richard Taylor (New York: Promethean Books, 1990).

FREQUENCY

Everybody wants to think of themselves as "normal," especially males who seem to need to compare and compete. So I am not surprised when I get this type of question.

Dear Sue: *How often do most couples have sex?*

Sue says: For starters, you need to know that in the United States the frequency of sexual activity has decreased in the past ten years. A decade ago, research shows, couples had sex 2.2 times a week. Today, couples are TTFS (Too Tired For Sex) or DINTFS (Double Income, No Time For Sex), and now they have sex once a week if they are lucky. The same study told us that most couples had sex Saturday nights or Sunday mornings and seldom had "nooners" or little "afternoon delights."

Frequency of sexual activity can depend on the stage of the relationship. When you are just falling in love, the intimacy is at its highest, and so is the excitement. You just can't get enough of it. You neck on the bus, you climb all over each other, and sex is to die for. That is the mad, passionate phase, which some people call "lust and limerance" and it lasts for approximately six months.

Then it simmers down and you move into compassionate love. Not as exciting but often more meaningful, comfortable, and satisfying. That's the way it's gonna be, with flashes of the old passion—wet, wild, wonderful, and worth the wait.

Couples who experience differences in their levels of desire need to develop good communication skills so that they both feel free to express their feelings without fear that they will be misinterpreted. And you have to be open to your partner's sexual cues—a wink, a nudge, a pat, or "you want to?" as well as being able to indicate "no go" without it being seen as rejection or a put-down.

If you feel like you hunger for sex less frequently than others, keep in mind that many men and women want sex not because they are genuinely horny, but to meet other needs, which might include:

- Reassurance that he/she can still do it, he/she is all man/woman.
- Hopes to keep the partner from wanting outside affairs. Frequency does not assure fidelity. One caller told me he had regular satisfying sex with his wife, but every morning on his way to work, he had a standing appointment with a prostitute for a blow job in his car.
- Loneliness, boredom, depression, or procrastination. (It sure beats scrubbing the kitchen floor!)

Dear Sue: *My boyfriend and I both love sex, wake each other up all night long, have sex a couple of times before work, during our lunch break, and when we get home from work. We have sex in public toilets, in movie theaters, on airplanes, in canoes, and under the dining-room table. Is it normal to have sex twenty-one times a day?*

Sue says. Now, does that make the rest of us feel inadequate or what? Just thinking about this is exhausting! But if both partners agree, if there is no manipulation, coercion, or exploitation, if that is what you both want, it is good, clean, if wet, fun. GO FOR IT.

Here's an interesting situation:

Dear Sue: *What's wrong with my partner? She never wants to have sex. She doesn't care if we never do it. I have tried everything, romantic weekends, wine, gifts, the whole bit, but it's no go. She used to love sex. What has happened?*

Sue says: We need to look at who has the problem here. She may be fine. She doesn't seem to be suffering from the lack of sex, but it sounds like you sure are. First step, you need to own the problem. You are responsible for your own sexual satisfaction. If your partner is not willing and able, you can simply masturbate and enjoy that. Neither of you should feel badly about that.

We need to understand that, like the appetite for food, some people have big appetites for sex and need lots of it; others need only small amounts, enough to keep body and soul together. And as with one's appetite for food, sexual appetite is not static; it changes. You may want to "pig out" for a period of time, but at another time you feel satiated with smaller amounts. This is not a problem in a good, open, communicating relationship. You can talk about it, understand your partner, and compromise. One would hope you would discover whether you are on the same sexual wavelength before you really get into a relationship.

The two of you, and your relationship, would benefit from good counseling. The therapist would want to rule out the possibility that sex was painful for her, and find out if she is using a good method of contraception. There is also the possibility that she was sexually assaulted when she was younger and is now suffering flashbacks.

You might be interested to hear that at one time I was inundated with letters from women who said that their husbands no longer wanted to have sex. Interestingly, women always blame themselves when this happens—they think he does not love them anymore, that they are not sexy enough, and that he has fallen in love with somebody else.

Although I receive fewer of these letters now, I still get a fair number of them:

Dear Sue: *The only time my husband ever touches me is when he wants sex. I ask for a hug and I get felt up, so I avoid all contact.*

Sue says: This is sad. We all need body contact, warm soft loving hugs, snuggles, pats, and stroking with no sexual overtones. Just warm "fuzzie-wuzzies."

Explain to your partner that you miss the feeling of closeness that comes from an affectionate hug and you are aware that this is just not happening now. Then both of you need to agree on sexual cues that will give you a very clear message of what the other person would like. And once your guard is down, you may be surprised how often you end up having great sex that just happened.

FUN SEX

Remember when you were courting and first married? Sex was fun, a romp, a lark in the park. After a while, it became monotonous, repetitious, Dullsville.

Dear Sue: *What can you do to spice up a boring sex life?*

Sue says: Besides sharing and implementing the fantasies you and your partner have, here are a few stunts that do not take a great deal of time and planning.

- Put a "mash" note in your partner's briefcase or lunch bag. ("I can't wait until you get home! I just want to jump your bones.")
- Buy a new fun sex toy, scented oil, a vibrator.
- Finger-paint each other's body on a big sheet on the floor.
- Go skinny-dipping together in the moonlight.
- Revisit the parking spot where you used to neck and make out.
- Celebrate the different seasons by making love in a

pile of leaves in the fall, in front of a fire in the winter, in a sleeping bag on the trail in spring, or on the beach in summer.

- Draft a love message by cutting the words or letters from newspapers and magazines.
- Make a special Saturday-morning candlelight breakfast with champagne and orange juice.
- If your partner is bashful or reluctant, get the revised edition of the old but good book *The Joy of Sex* by Dr. Alex Comfort (New York: Crown, 2002), rev. ed., or *Light Her Fire* by Ellen Kreidman (New York: Dell, 1992), *Urge: Hot Secrets for Great Sex* by Dr. Gabrielle Morrissey (Boston: Thorsons, 2003), *The Good Orgasm Guide* by Kate Taylor (New York: Barnes & Noble, 2003), *Tricks to Please a Woman* by Jay Wiseman (San Francisco: Greenery Press, 2002), or *Seduce Me: How to Ignite Your Partner's Passion* by Darcy A. Cole (Booklocker.com, 2003).

[g]

G-SPOT

If I do a segment on the G-spot on my radio show or on TV, I know I will receive a deluge of mail for the next two weeks.

From a guy:

Dear Sue: Thank God you talked about the G-spot. It sure changed my girlfriend's interest in hot sex. She used to love sex and could really get into it, but then one night she spurted all this fluid, literally quarts of it, all over me and the bed. She couldn't stop it. She said it was "the best." We did not know what happened, but she decided she must have peed in the bed. She was so embarrassed that she would hold back for fear that it would happen again. Personally, I didn't care. After all, it was her bed. Please tell us more about this spot and how come I have never heard about it before.

Sue says: What a comment on our times, when the most glorious sexual experience can, because of lack of information, make us feel guilty, ashamed, embarrassed, and abnormal—so much so that we swear it will never happen again.

Women who have experienced the G-spot orgasm tell me it is the ultimate in "wet sex." It seems to happen when a woman is very relaxed, comfortable with her body, and really into pleasure—she doesn't care how she looks, sounds, or smells; she is very, very sexually aroused and has already had one or two orgasms.

It appears to happen more often to women who have had a baby because they know what it is like to really "bear down." While her partner continues to stimulate her, she takes a deep breath and pushes. Suddenly all this fluid comes gushing out. And there is a lot of it, like liters. Guys have told me they thought a dam had burst. One guy thought his lover would drown him because she was holding his head "down there" and wouldn't let him up for air.

At the end of all this, a woman feels invigorated and happy, but limp, with no energy, like a rag doll with a silly grin on her face.

The G-spot is named after a Dr. Grafenburg. Now, the medical term for a G-spot orgasm is "orgasmic expulsion." There is still not a great deal of information available simply because experts are unable to pinpoint and label the area, nor can they locate the nerves that trigger the response. Researchers believe that there is a patch of erectile tissue inside the vagina, which, when stimulated, results in fluid collecting in the bladder. When a woman pushes or bears down, the fluid spurts out through the urethra.

It is definitely *not* urine. It smells sweet, like freshly cut hay, and does not stain the mattress as urine does, although the sheets dry stiff. The components of the fluid are different from the composition of urine.

I have heard some pretty funny stories about the G-spot. One couple rigged up an electric hair dryer aimed at the wet spot because they found it took at least a week for the mattress to dry out. Another woman had an electric heater topple over and set fire to the mattress. Imagine trying to explain that to the firefighters who arrived carrying axes. My theory is, always do it on his side of the bed.

Do take a look at *Seduce Me: How to Ignite Your Partner's Passion* by Darcy A. Cole (Booklocker.com, 2003).

But there could be trouble in paradise:

Dear Sue: *I am really frustrated because my boyfriend will stop sex before I reach orgasm simply because I hit the G-spot and he is fed up with having a wet mattress all the time.*

Sue says: I like to use Rational Emotive Therapy with problems like this. Your initial gut reaction (mine, too) is to say, "Well, forget it big boy, you ain't gonna get none." And that would work. You'd make your point, but you would probably be throwing the baby out with the bathwater and the relationship could end. So if that's not what you want, then try this very practical solution.

Take a big green garbage bag, cut along one side and across the top, and open it up. Pin the four corners of a huge bath towel or flannelette sheet to the four corners of the plastic. Roll it up and put it under the bed. Now, when things start to get hot, you make a big production of whipping this bedroll out, and place it under you, from your hips to your toes, 'cause you're gonna need it. (You can always hang it over the railing of the balcony to dry and make the neighbors jealous.) If this ritual is going to be repeated frequently, why not invest in a waterbed with a plastic mattress? Then you'd only end up with wet sheets. Hey, it's worth it.

Whatever you do, you need to talk to him, tell him how you feel (put down, angry, cheated, frustrated). If this relationship is going to continue, then you want to be able to enjoy sex as much as he does—wet spot and all.

The G-spot is receiving some exposure on various talk shows, and as a result, I get another kind of letter.

Dear Sue: *How can I locate my girlfriend's G-spot? She used to hit it all the time with her ex-boyfriend, but I can't find it.*

Sue says: I am concerned that you are becoming goal-oriented, and that your new bottom line is the G-spot. If you continue this way, sex will not be for pleasure but to prove that you are as good a lover as her ex. Are you putting this pressure on yourself, or is she taunting and making you feel inadequate? If so, we have to look at whether she is playing a game for power and control in your relationship.

Performance anxiety will affect pleasure and enjoyment for both of you, and if you feel you have failed, you may give up on sex. Talk about it with your girlfriend. Tell her how you feel; ask her to guide you to what pleases her, and then relax and enjoy. While the G-spot is a nice bonus, it is not essential. Many, many females never get there and are perfectly happy and contented. So please do not make it your only purpose for sex. If it happens, wonderful, and if not, well, maybe it will another time.

Some women can bring themselves to G-spot orgasm by masturbating and stimulating the clitoris and the inside of the vagina with one hand and pushing down on their abdomen just above their pubic bone with the other.

For more information on orgasmic expulsion, please pick up the paperback entitled *The Good Vibrations Guide: The G Spot* by Cathy Winks (San Francisco: Down There Press, 1998).

GENDER SELECTION

Most couples pay lip service to the idea, "We don't care whether it is a boy or a girl as long as it's healthy." But they secretly fantasize about the perfect "millionaire's family"—a boy first, to carry on the family name and/or business, then two or three years later, a beautiful feminine baby girl for Mommy to fuss over. In some cultures, having a male child is essential for looking after the parents in their old age and to work the fields. In urban China, there are strict limits on family size—one child only. Male babies are preferred. In such cultures there is strong pressure on a wife to have a male child. Even though the sex of a baby is determined by the chromosomes in the father's ejaculate, the mother is blamed if she does not have a son. In North America, a situation such as this one is very common:

Dear Sue: My wife and I have three boys and we are willing to try again if we can be assured that we will have a girl.

Sue says: There are so many theories about choosing the sex of your baby. Supposedly, sperm carrying the Y chromosome (male) are heavier and travel faster than the lighter, slower, and more lasting X chromosome. So if you want a boy, have sex early in the ovulatory cycle. At this point, the Y chromosome will have gone rushing headlong through and reached the egg first, so you will have a better chance for a boy. If you want a girl, have sex two or three days before the egg is released. By the time of ovulation, the Y sperm have gone ahead, found nobody home, and they died; the slower, more resilient X chromosome (female) will fertilize the egg. Lotsa luck. Honestly.

A recent study found that assertive, self-reliant women have a higher testosterone level and are also more likely to conceive sons. Researchers believe the higher hormone level makes an egg reject X-sperm and accept Y (male)-sperm. Because stress and other factors influence testosterone levels, women with average levels may vary enough to conceive both boys and girls. If a woman's levels are always high, however, she might have an all-boy family. This puts a whole new spin on gender selection.

One old wives' tale instructs douching with a weak vinegar solution two hours after sex if you want a boy. The sperm carrying the Y (male) chromosome will already be there, and you will kill off all the slower X (female) chromosomes. Myth. And you'll end up with a "pickled vagina" to boot.

A little more scientific and a lot more expensive are the gender-selection services. There, doctors filter the heavier Y chromosomes out of the ejaculate and artificially inseminate the woman when she is ovulating. It will probably take three separate attempts, each costing more than six hundred dollars. This service is not covered by any medical plan, and there are no money-back guarantees.

In cultures where is strong pressure on a wife to have a male child, couples who are desperate to have a baby of a particular gender may resort to using the service of unscrupulous gynecologists who wait until the mother is about fourteen weeks pregnant, at which point they do an amniocentesis or ultrasound to determine the gender of the fetus. If the baby is the wrong gender, they immediately do a therapeutic abortion.

In our communities we must support women by removing

the stigma placed on them if they do not produce a son, and we can work toward changing attitudes that place more importance on male children than female. Moreover, we must provide equal opportunities in education for both of them.

GUILT

Everyone experiences guilt at some time in life. Guilt is what you feel when you follow a "want" that goes against one of your "shoulds." You do something that you believe to be wrong. The guilt feeling is worse if you are caught and made to feel unworthy, ashamed, or that you cannot be trusted in the future.

Women seem to be more susceptible to guilt than men. The wonderful one-liner "Show me a woman who does not feel guilty and I'll show you a man" may be true. Women can "should" themselves to death!

Your attitudes and values, what you believe is right or wrong, were established by age ten. Your parents, siblings, grandparents, school, church, and peers all influenced your concept of what was acceptable and unacceptable behavior.

You spent your teen years gathering more information, looking at your attitudes and values, trying out different behaviors, and finding which ones fit into your concept of what life was all about. You shared and compared your ideas with your peers. You established your "oughts and shoulds" and chose guidelines by which to live.

It is amazing, but you will not change these values until there is a crisis in your life that forces you to rethink your values. This letter is a classic example:

Dear Sue: This load of guilt is the only glitch on my horizon of happiness. When I was twenty, I was engaged to my won-

derful boyfriend. But one evening he was away and I went to a party, had too much to drink, and had quickie sex in the bathroom with another guy. I got pregnant. I think that guy is the father. My boyfriend, thinking the baby was his, married me. My son is now eight and a really good kid, but every time I look at him, I think of my awful secret. The guilt is affecting my relationship with my husband and our son. I keep wondering if I would feel better if I told all. What do you think?

Sue says: There are some effective ways of handling guilt. Look at what you did and think honestly about why you did it. What were your motives? Were they valid and realistic? Did you accomplish what you had hoped? If you did, but you still feel guilty because you hurt somebody else in the process or you really went against all that you believe in, then it might be beneficial to seek short-term counseling from a qualified counselor/therapist.

See a doctor, psychologist, psychiatrist, marriage counselor, or sex therapist to help you work through guilt. In some instances, talking to a good friend can be beneficial, providing you know that confidentiality will be guaranteed. But if your friend does not respect your request for confidentiality, she might betray your confidence. It could be devastating if the truth accidentally leaked out. So I would be reluctant to tell anybody about your problem other than a professional.

In the case of any indiscretion, before you get into true confessions with your partner, think seriously about why you want to "tell all."

Many times confessions like this are an attempt to dump the guilt onto your partner and absolve yourself: "I did the right thing. I told him about the truth—how he reacts is his problem."

It is also important to be aware of your partner's attitudes and values. Would he ever be able to forgive you? Would he ever trust you again? Would your confession act as a catalyst to get the relationship back on track? Or would it be the last straw? Be sure you know what you are doing and why you are doing it. Something to think about: no one can make you feel guilty without your permission.

It's a myth that there should be no secrets between partners. In reality, there are some things that are best left unshared. There is wisdom in the old adage "A little knowledge can be a dangerous thing." You will have to consider all the possible ramifications of disclosure.

There are ways of coping with guilt that are nonproductive and even harmful to yourself and to others:

- You may ignore the guilty feelings and try to suppress them or deny that they are there. The more you try, the more you become preoccupied with the feelings of guilt. That, combined with the fear that your secret will be discovered, can result in your becoming uncommunicative and withdrawn.
- You may try to escape by blaming someone else or the circumstances.
- You may try to drown the feelings with drugs or alcohol, tranquilizers or sleeping pills.
- You may devote your time to trying to atone for your actions, to make up for them, to earn forgiveness.
- You may decide to severely restrict your behavior in an effort to prevent the same thing from ever happening again, or to prove to others that you have learned your lesson and it will never happen again. This knee-jerk reaction will not remove the guilt but will affect your self-concept and self-esteem.

- You may act in a way that harms your relationship with the people you feel guilty about. Which would hurt those relationships the most: the truth, hiding the truth, or your guilt?

If you can really examine what you did and why you did it, and why you are feeling guilty, you can decide if the guilt has been imposed on you by other people to control your behavior. Feelings of remorse and regret for a foolish mistake are honest reactions.

Keep a journal of your feelings. Write them down—you do not have to justify them. When you reread them in six months, a clear picture will emerge. Then you will be more focused if you decide to discuss your behavior with the other person. You will be able to express regret and remorse and be free of the controlling guilt.

If the other person simply refuses to let go, insists on trying to control you by making you feel guilty, then that individual has the problem. Do not allow yourself to get hooked into someone else's game.

When other people realize that they can no longer control you by applying generous quantities of guilt, perhaps they will give up that game plan, and perhaps you can establish an egalitarian relationship. If not, you may have to give up the relationship and move on with your life.

Guilt is a self-administered punishment imposed by yourself or somebody else when you are convinced you have violated values imposed by society. It can be destructive, so it is important to work to eliminate guilt from your life.

[h]

HAIRINESS

Dear Sue: *I am twenty years old, a single female, and I have a mustache on my upper lip. I also have hairy nipples and my pubic hair grows down my thighs. This is not appealing. I have tried shaving, plucking, and waxing. Bleaching just gives me a blond fuzzy appearance. This is just too much for electrolysis. I feel like Godzilla. Anything I can do?*

Sue says: In some races, both males and females are more prone to developing body hair. It is called hirsutism. Go to your family doctor for an extensive family-history analysis. If your hirsutism is not hereditary, the doctor may refer you to an endocrinologist, a doctor who specializes in hormones, who will test your hormone levels. You may have a high testosterone reading, which has resulted in excess body hair.

There is also a drug called spironolactone, which could be helpful. It is available by prescription only. Check with your doctor.

We have always been told that shaving makes the hair grow in thicker, coarser, and faster. Recent research seems to indicate that this is not true.

An interesting aside—they say that sailors out at sea for long periods notice their beards do not grow nearly as fast as when they are in port and in the presence of women.

HEADACHE

Dear Sue: *We all laugh when we hear the excuse "Not tonight, dear, I've got a headache." But it is not funny if it happens all the time. Could these headaches be for real?*

Sue says: It's not funny for either partner, whether the headaches are real or fabricated.

If your partner has genuine headaches frequently, we need to find the cause and see if there is a cure or prevention. Headaches can be caused by factors that range from stress, allergies, fatigue, and eyestrain to more serious (and less common) illnesses. Headache treatments are as diverse as these causes, from painkillers to yoga and acupuncture.

Turns out, sex may even serve as a headache treatment. An American study showed that about one third to one half of women who had sex when they had a headache found orgasm relieved the pain. The theory is that vaginal stimulation released an analgesic substance that cured or alleviated the headache. There could be a new twist to "I have a headache"—she snuggles up to her partner and says, "Honey, help me cure it."

Also, many women have found masturbation relieves headaches. Would that be a possibility she might consider? We also know that females masturbate to eliminate menstruation cramps. Never underestimate the power of sex!

If your partner's headaches are an excuse to avoid sex, it would be in the category with "I'm too tired," or "The baby will hear us," or "I have my period" for the second time this month. The funniest one I have heard is a woman who used to rub Vicks VapoRub all over her nose and chest, knowing her husband would not come near her.

If your partner's headaches fall into this category, we have to find out what is going on in the relationship. Is there unresolved conflict or anger? Is she expressing the need for power and control or getting even and punishing you for some injustice?

Women do not have a monopoly on headaches. Because more females are initiating sex, males, who for generations have complained, "It would be nice if, just once, she made the first move," are now backpedaling when she does make a move. Same old lines: fatigue, stress, too much to drink, or "nobody's home down there."

Occasionally, both males and females may develop a splitting headache that may last for hours or days after sex. Sexual arousal causes blood vessels to dilate and there is an increase of blood supply to the genitals, so that less goes to the brain. Lack of oxygen produces pain similar to a migraine. After sex, circulation returns to normal and the headache settles into a dull throbbing. Do see your doctor if this happens.

If there is nausea, vomiting, weakness, or numbness, see your doctor without delay. Go to the emergency room if you have an explosive headache of blinding intensity. This could be a blood vessel or aneurysm rupturing, and although they are uncommon, they are two very serious possibilities.

HOMOSEXUALITY

The lesbian and gay community have a slogan: "We're queer, we're here, get used to it." But our society is having difficulty accepting homosexuality even though it is estimated that anywhere between 2 and 10 percent of our male population is gay, and between 1 and 4 percent of females are lesbians.

Parents want to be good parents with the perfect *Leave It to Beaver* family. They share and compare with other parents, looking for indications that their kids are normal, if not above average, and are devastated if they are perceived as "different."

I would like to encourage people to learn all they can about homosexuality so we can reduce, or preferably eliminate, the bias some people feel against gays. If parents did not talk about homosexuality in a derogatory way, using such terms as "queer," "pansy," and "lezzie," there would be more acceptance and humanity. Schools would do well to have the topic included in their sex-education curriculum in order to reduce homophobia. Do read *Is It a Choice? Answers to 300 of the Most Commonly Asked Questions About Gays and Lesbians* by Eric Marcus (San Francisco: HarperSanFrancisco, 1999), rev. ed., and *How to Be a Happy Lesbian: A Coming Out Guide* by Tracey Stevens and Katherine Wunder (Asheville: Amazing Dreams Publishing, 2002).

Dear Sue: *I am really worried about my five-year-old son. He is a sissy. He prefers dolls to trucks. He dances and prances when other kids are tearing around. He doesn't yell, he* *squeals. He is so "femme" that I am embarrassed when we go to family celebrations. Am I raising him to be gay? Is there anything I can do to straighten him out?*

Sue says: He's five years old! What boy is macho at that age, and why would you want him to be? Don't even think about trying to remake your son. It will not work and you will only manage to mess him up totally. You are *not* making him gay. Let's get some information here. I sincerely hope you will learn to relax, and accept and enjoy your magnificent son.

We do not know what "causes" homosexuality. We used to believe if a boy had a strong mother and a weak father, he would mimic mother and reject male stereotypes; on the other hand, if a boy had a strong father and a weak mother, son identifies with father. Not so.

Then researchers reasoned that a male who was "different" lacked male sex hormones, so they gave him injections of testosterone, and guess what? He became more effeminate. The next theory was that homosexuality was a psychiatric disorder. So they tried behavior modification and aversion therapy, a treatment that was also unsuccessful. Religious fundamentalists still insist that homosexuals can reverse their sexual orientation if they "accept God."

Recent research indicates that the hypothalamus (a small, round gland located at the base of the brain, which regulates many body systems) in a gay male's brain is very similar to that of a female. No research has been done on the brains of lesbians. Also, it does appear that homosexuality runs in families, usually on the mother's side. It is not uncommon that two or three or all the children in a family are gay or lesbian. But this has not been well documented yet.

Personally, I do not care what "causes" homosexuality—

that implies it is abnormal. For a gay person, it is no more abnormal than having blond hair and blue eyes. Trying to find a cause also implies that we should be trying to "cure homosexuality," but most lesbians and gays do not want to be "cured." They want acceptance by society and freedom to develop as individuals, without fear or rejection and recrimination. Isn't that what we all want—the four big *A*s: acceptance, approval, appreciation, and attention?

If he is gay, society, school, and the world will all be very hard for your son to deal with until he is an adult and has developed coping skills and found a community where he is comfortable. He is going to need all the love and support that you as parents can give.

Many parents, antennae up, watch a child like this develop, and when the boy is about three, they become suspicious but say nothing, subtly attempting to steer him to more "gender-appropriate" activities and friends. At about age six, kids themselves feel "different" but are unable to tell what is unusual. By age ten their friends are snickering about girls and "boobies" and sometimes they sneak a peek at *Playboy,* but he is just not interested in girls. He may make the appropriate heterosexual jokes and make passes at girls. If he is extremely effeminate, he will be teased and ostracized by the other boys. The girls will like him, though, because he is "not a jerk like the other guys." Unfortunately, this leaves him vulnerable to being roughed up by other guys. Early on, he may have his first experiences of gay bashing.

By age fourteen he becomes very aware that he is not attracted to females, but he does become aroused when he fantasizes about sex with other males. In all probability, he is still very much "in the closet"; it is just too risky to "come out" to anybody.

If he grows up in or moves to a large city, he will find the gay community, where he will meet a group of lesbians and gays with whom he can be comfortable, dating and experimenting with sex. Many guys who are attracted to other men have sex with females just to try it out and compare, and then they know. This is why sex education and Safer Sex messages must be made available early.

By his late teens, a guy realizes he is homosexual but may not be ready to disclose this to his parents. However, he may tell a few close friends. Only when he leaves home and perhaps has a lover will he come to terms with his homosexuality.

Some parents feel it is essential that they push him: "When are you gonna get a girlfriend? Why don't you take out that nice girl you met at church?"

One hopes that parents will be able to show love and support so that their child's coming out will not be a painful process. There is a wonderful organization called Parents and Friends of Lesbians and Gays (P-FLAG) that provides information and support for families of people who are homosexual. They can be reached at 1726 M St. NW, Suite 400, Washington, DC 20036; phone 202-467-8180; fax 202-467-8194; www.pflag.org.

Can you imagine the angst of the young male who wrote the following letter?

Dear Sue: *I am a fifteen-year-old boy and I am terrified that I might be gay. I am totally unable to get an erection with girls, although I like them as best friends. I fantasize about sex with older boys. I've been called "femme" and "swishy." My family laughs and yammers at me to act like a man. There is no way I can live as a queer. I want to be a politician, and no one would elect a fag. I want to be normal, get married, and have a family. Tell me I'm not gay.*

Sue says: At fifteen you just cannot be absolutely certain of your sexual orientation, and I would hope you could just let it be for a while. This is not something you have to decide on by midnight tonight. When the time comes, it will all be clear, and you will know. Do not label yourself as homosexual until you are very sure.

Fearing you are gay or being labeled a homosexual in high school can be disastrous. Kids ostracize you, tease you, and can even be violent. This is tough to deal with in tenth grade. The statistics are pretty scary. Ten percent of all kids attempt suicide, and of those, one third do so because they are concerned about their sexual orientation.

So you really do need to find somebody you can trust to talk to. Perhaps your family doctor, a guidance counselor or teacher to whom you can relate, or a school nurse, a minister, or someone in your family whom you know to be "gay positive." If you feel you just cannot rely on their support, look in the phone book and find any gay and lesbian counseling service. These services are free and confidential, and the people will not lecture, preach, or try to change you.

Dear Sue: *With all the homophobia out there today, why would anybody choose to be gay?*

Sue says: Simple. You do not choose your sexual orientation. You just are gay or straight or bi. Stop and think. At what stage of your life did you sit down and decide, "Well, I think I will be attracted to the opposite sex." You didn't. You just knew. At puberty, your hormones kicked in and suddenly you had a crush on a rock star of the opposite sex, or one of the same sex. Having an occasional erotic dream or fantasizing about somebody of the same sex does not mean you are homosexual. It means you are normal.

Dear Sue: *Homosexuality does not bother me, but I sure get uncomfortable when I see them on the subway kissing. Why do they flaunt it in public?*

Sue says: Great question. Why does anybody show affection in public?

- To show the world that they are in love and what the whole world thinks does not matter one iota.
- Because they feel passionately about each other and can't get enough of each other, which happens in the hetero world, too.
- To make a public statement about their sexual orientation as a form of defiance, flaunting it, rubbing your nose in it.

Would you feel the same way if they were a heterosexual couple necking and petting on the subway? In all probability, you would. We are taught that public displays of affection are inappropriate, because these feelings are personal and private.

What would you do if they were hetero? Probably you would frown and look away. I doubt your disapproval would discourage a hetero couple, nor would it affect a homosexual couple, so ignore it or move to a different seat in the subway car.

Dear Sue: *What is a "lipstick dyke"?*

Sue says: Lesbians are taking back their language and acting proud. More and more, lesbians will, without reservation, call themselves dyke, butch dyke, bitch dyke. No problem. It is the hetero community who regards being called a dyke as a put-down, a slam at femininity, or a lack a lack of it, so *we* have the problem. I have never called anybody "dyke" in the same way that I would never call anybody "fag." I would feel they might interpret it as a put-down because I am hetero, Although it is okay for them to refer to themselves that way, I would not feel comfortable using that language.

A lipstick lesbian is a very attractive, well-dressed, sexy female who does not look like the stereotypical lesbian (short hair, work boots, plaid shirt).

Other lesbians feel that the reason for wearing makeup is to attract males, and they are not out to attract males. Lipstick lesbians say they feel they look better with makeup. Two sides of the same coin.

A teenage female can be a tomboy, can wear grunge clothes, and not be labeled as lesbian unless she is open about her attraction to other females. As an adult, she can flaunt being a "dyke." While her parents may not be overjoyed, nobody makes her life difficult. However, as a teen she may have difficulty finding another female her age to date. Some females are very sure during adolescence that they are lesbian, but most women have matured and may be married and have children before they come to accept it.

Dear Sue: *Peggy and I have been a couple for nine years. We are both professionals, own our own home, and have an active social life—all heterosexual. Both of us are "in the closet" at work—nobody knows we are lesbians. Would it damage our careers if we came out to friends and coworkers?*

Sue says: This is a very personal choice, which you should make together after some serious discussion. Many in the lesbian and gay community are adamant and vocal in their conviction that homosexuals have an obligation to go public with their sexual preference. By remaining in the closet, they believe, you are feeding into the myth that homosexuals are "different" or a threat to family values.

Some homosexuals maintain that you can't be a whole person while denying that aspect of yourself. On the other hand, most gays and lesbians have experienced rejection and prejudice. As a result, they are so aware of the prevailing homophobia that some have decided that their sexual orientation is no one else's business and have kept it under wraps to avoid hassles.

Only you can decide if coming out would jeopardize your career. You can be selective about whom you decide to come out to. Think about it carefully—it is easier to do than to undo.

Dear Sue: *I have been married for four years. Shortly after our baby was born, I had the feeling my husband was having an affair. My brother followed him one night when he went out with the boys. Yeah, out with the boys was right. He went to a gay bar, cruised and schmoozed for a while, then went to some guy's apartment. Is he some kind of homo or something?*

Sue says: Before you jump to conclusions, can you trust your brother? Does he dislike your husband? Would your brother make up a story that would upset and/or annoy you? If you can really believe him, don't jump to conclusions—you still do not know for sure what went on in that apartment. Be very calm and collected. Do not blame and do not accuse your husband. Simply tell him what you are concerned about and what you know for sure. (It's best to leave your brother out of it.) Then listen—really listen. When he is finished explaining, tell him you are upset and you need time to think about this.

Do not allow him to sweep you off your feet with sweet talk, and do *not* have unprotected sex with him. If he lies about going out with his friends, you have an obligation to yourself and to your baby.

You must practice Safer Sex. And if he does not accept that, then you can put him on "couch patrol" until you are 101 percent convinced that you are not at risk. This is your life. Do not jeopardize it just to keep him happy.

There are some great books and videos about homosexuality that will give you more information and reassurances that gay is good: *Loving Someone Gay* by Don Clark (Berkeley: Celestial Arts, 1997); *Is It a Choice? Answers to 300 of the Most Commonly Asked Questions about Gays and Lesbians* by Eric Marcus (San Francisco: HarperSanFrancisco, 1999), rev. ed.; *The Ins and Outs of Gay Sex* by Stephen E. Goldstone (New York: Dell, 1999); *The Whole Lesbian Sex Book* by Felice Newman (San Francisco: Cleis, 1999); *GLBTQ: The Survival Guide for Queer and Questioning Teens* by Kelly Huegel (Minneapolis: Free Spirit, 2003).

HYSTERECTOMY

Dear Sue: My doctor has referred me to a gynecologist with the recommendation that I have a hysterectomy. What does this mean?

Sue says: A hysterectomy is the surgical removal of part or all of the female reproductive system. If a woman has cancer of the uterus, the cervix, uterus, fallopian tubes, and ovaries are removed. (The ovaries are removed because hormones from the ovaries can exacerbate cancerous growths.) This type of surgery is called a bilateral salpingoophorectomy and hysterectomy. This operation is also performed if the woman has extensive endometriosis, uterine fibroids, or a prolapsed uterus.

In most hysterectomies performed today, the uterus and cervix are removed and the ovaries and the distal ends of the fallopian tubes are left intact. This means you do not go through surgical menopause. In either instance, the top of the vagina is closed off to become a dead-end street.

Dear Sue: *My doctor is recommending I have a hysterectomy because I have benign fibroids and "periods from hell." I practically hemorrhage for two weeks of every month. I am so scared. Will I be normal again?*

Sue says: Are you normal now, "flooding" for fourteen out of twenty-eight days? What's normal to you? If by this you mean can you get pregnant and carry a baby to term, you will not be able to do this after a hysterectomy. But will you feel, look, and act sexy? Yes, and more so because you will not spend half your life with mattress-size sanitary pads between your legs.

Let's address the major myth surrounding hysterectomy: you will not be a "complete woman" after the operation. False. Many women will tell you that after their hysterectomy, they had a new lease on life. Because they no longer have a cervix, they have no concerns about Pap smears or cancer of the cervix. They have energy to burn because their hemoglobin count has gone way up, they've been freed from monthly periods and fear of pregnancy, and some have told me that they've become enthusiastic about sex for the first time in years.

Menopause is one side effect for women who have hysterectomies in which the ovaries are removed. If you still have your ovaries, you will produce estrogen and progesterone, so you will not go through menopause immediately;

although it will start earlier than usual, it will be gradual. Unless you have cancer, you can go on hormone replacement therapy (HRT) to ease difficulties during menopause. Because you do not have a uterus, you will not need progesterone, just estrogen. During menopause, if you find your vaginal walls become dry and irritated and tear easily, you would benefit from applying estrogen cream to your labia and vaginal walls daily.

There are some tragic stories, such as the following:

Dear Sue: *I was thirty-seven when I had a hysterectomy, everything out. The doctors, the nurses, nobody told me a thing. I crashed. Not only did I feel depressed, but I became "loony tunes" with my family, had hot flashes, night sweats, headaches, the whole scene. I kept going back to the doctor, but he did nothing. Finally, I went to another doctor and was given a prescription for hormone replacement therapy, and it was instant turnaround. I have never felt better.*

Dear Sue: *Will my husband be aware of any changes if I have a hysterectomy?*

Sue says: In terms of his sexual pleasure and satisfaction, *no*. The vagina may be slightly shorter but can still contain his penis, and because your cervix has been removed, his penis will not be banging up against it. That could feel better for both of you. But you will not be gender neuter or asexual.

Now, it may take as long as a year to get your full, roaring sex drive back, not because of the surgery but because your hormone balance will be thrown out of whack. You may notice a change in the deep sensation of orgasm as a result of loss of uterine contractions. Some women really enjoy sex, "no holds barred," postoperatively.

Some doctors tell their patients to wait for as long as six weeks for healing to be complete, and until after the postoperative checkup before resuming intercourse. But if you are in a stable relationship, where there is no possibility of STIs, and your partner is gentle, tender, and caring, then you can try intercourse as soon as you feel that it is what you want. The operative words here are "gently, Bentley."

But let's be honest, if you did not enjoy sex before surgery, then a hysterectomy will not turn you into a sexpot overnight.

Some good books: *Hysterectomy and the Alternatives* by Jan Clark (New York: Vintage, 2000); *The Gynecological Sourcebook* by M. Sara Rosenthal (New York: McGraw-Hill, 2003), 4th ed.

[i]

IMPOTENCE (ERECTILE DYSFUNCTION)

Dear Sue: *My husband of twenty-five years is no longer able to get an erection so that we can have sex. I have heard great things about Viagra. Tell me more*

Sue says: Viagra has been available by prescription from your family doctor, and although it is a little expensive, it works for most men. It works by allowing the blood to flow into the penis and stay there for a couple of hours. That should do it, eh? Now, for it to be effective, he must be interested in sex, ready for sex, aroused, and receptive. He would take one blue pill, and it takes about twenty minutes to work—plenty of time to woo you and stimulate you so that you are aroused, too.

Men who are on any heart medication are not candidates for Viagra. Some males have complained of visual disturbances—they see a blue aura—and others may get a severe headache or digestive upsets. But on the whole, it is safe. The only complication occurs if the erection does not subside after a few hours, in which case a man must go to the hospital.

Viagra is invaluable in a loving, caring relationship, for both parties must consider intercourse to be an integral component of their relationship. Where we have trouble in paradise is if the couple has not been able to talk about the "problem," share their feelings, and agree they want to try Viagra. Some women never liked sex in the first place, and now that he has this erectile dysfunction, they are glad not to feel they "should" have sex to keep him satisfied—and now he expects it again. Now that he's found Viagra, some women feel that they should participate in sex or he will go out on the prowl, looking for another partner who is more enthusiastic. Also, if he was a lousy, inconsiderate lover before he developed erectile dysfunction, he will again be a lousy lover when he gets an erection. And some women blame themselves and feel inadequate that they were unable to turn him on enough to have an erection.

For these reasons I would prefer that the family doctor speak to the man and separately to his partner and do any necessary counseling.

There is another Viagra-type drug out, Cialis, which has fewer side effects. Check with your family doctor.

Here is a wonderful letter:

Dear Sue: *My husband is diabetic and has been impotent for years. He could satisfy me in other ways, but I missed the nice feelings of intercourse. So we tried everything. Some things worked, but most didn't and we gave up on all of them.*

Then an older doctor described "stuffing." We both enjoy tucking his penis (no erection) into my vagina. I can feel some throbbing. I don't know if it's him or me, but it feels great. We move our bodies in rhythm, in a thrusting or circular motion. For us, that is as good as it gets, and that is fine by us. Just thought I'd let you know.

Sue says: What more can I say but thanks.

INCEST

If there is any place in this world where young children should be safe, you would think it would be with their family. Unfortunately, statistics from both Canada and the United States tell us that one in four women and one in five men have been sexually abused at some stage of their life. Many researchers believe the statistics are higher, that victims simply do not disclose what happened. The long-term consequences are devastating.

Dear Sue: *When I was a little kid, I was molested by my father. My mother worked nights in a hospital. He would give me a bath, put me to bed, and crawl in beside me. He told me he was lonely, that he needed me and I made him feel better and I was not to tell anybody because they would not understand. He would touch me, stick his fingers into my vagina, get on top and come all over me, or make me take his huge penis in my mouth and shove my head the way he wanted it to go.*

I did not tell anybody, but I was so scared of my dad that I am sure my mom must have suspected. If she did, she never said a thing. I got an infection, and my doctor treated it, and he told my dad to lay off or he would call the authorities. Dad never touched me again and I left home as soon as I could.

The problem now is, I can't love anybody. I don't trust any-

body. I don't want to be touched by anybody and I feel like shit. You gotta help me.

Sue says: Okay, help is on the way. You have made a great start at helping yourself. You know what happened, you know what is causing your inability to relate to anybody on an intimate level, and you disclosed it to me. That tells me that you are now ready to make a move from victim to survivor. It will not be painless because there is so much trauma, betrayal, and distrust. It won't go away overnight, but you have made a great start. Just putting your recollections of the incest down on paper must have been very painful. It tells me you are one very strong lady, ready to start healing.

Make a plan of attack. The first move is to find a good counselor. Ask your doctor, or a rape crisis center. Any women's clinic or family-planning clinic should know of a few good counselors. You can also look in the phone book under "Marriage and Family Counseling" or under "Psychologists." If finances are a problem, ask your doctor to refer you to a psychiatrist.

It may take a few months to get your appointment, but you can start out on your own. You may find it helpful to keep a daily journal of feelings, reactions, and responses.

Write a long letter to your father, telling him exactly how you feel about what he did. Set the letter aside for a week and review and reassess before you decide whether to mail it. You need to write to your mother, too. She did not protect you as a parent should. Don't think about mailing these letters; just write, don't protect, excuse, or justify their behavior. There is *no* excuse for what happened. Tell your parents exactly what they did to you and how you feel. This is hard work—lotsa feelings, lotsa tears. Healing hurts. Then you can move on to the next phase, developing a good self-concept and high self-esteem, increasing your ability to trust, and getting a handle on the role of sex in your life.

Counseling and therapy are no quick and easy fix. It will take time and there may be regression, but hang in there. This is good work and you will come out a winner.

The long-term effects of this trauma, if untreated, can prevent you from ever living a normal, relatively happy, productive life. Some women bury the remembrance of abuse, but the effects manifest themselves in other ways such as depression, self-mutilation, severe headaches, avoidance of intimacy, flashbacks during a loving sexual relationship, and even attempted suicide. Some resort to drugs or alcohol as an escape.

Women who were victims of incest want to protect their children, so they supervise them and do not let them become independent. Or, the women may be harsh and detached in an attempt to prepare their children for the outside world and make them independent and self-sufficient at a young age.

False-memory syndrome is a new theory that maintains that memories are not accurate and that a manipulative therapist could lead a vulnerable client to untrue accusations. Do read *The Myth of Repressed Memory* by Dr. E. Loftus and K. Ketcham (New York: St. Martin's Press, 1994).

You may be able to find a support group for survivors of incest. Involvement in a group can provide support and convince you that you are not alone, that this is *not* your fault, and that you can get through it with a little help from your friends.

Women tell so many horror stories of incest, but males have also been sexually assaulted, occasionally by parents or by older siblings or other members of their extended family. Most often, males are assaulted by other older males who are friends of the family or well known to the victim.

It is more difficult to find good counseling for males who were sexually abused as children. There are few support groups, and few books specifically for them. However, I recommend these two books: *Victims No Longer: Men Recovering from Incest and Other Sexual Child Abuse* by Mike Lew (New York: Perennial, 1990); *Broken Boys—Mending Men: Recovery from Childhood Sexual Abuse* by Stephen D. Grubman-Black (West Caldwell: The Blackburn Press, 2002).

INCONTINENCE

Dear Sue: *Mygawd, I'm losing it completely. Ever since my babies (five of them) were born, I have had little "accidents" and would dribble urine, but I could always stop it. Now, at age fifty-three, I am finding that if I do aerobics, even low-impact stuff, or if I cough, laugh, or sneeze, I wet my pants and I can't stop. Is there anything I can do or shall I resign myself to wearing Pampers for the rest of my life?*

Sue says: This is called stress incontinence, and though it can happen to both sexes, it is more common among females. Women who have had babies, who have had repeated bladder infections, or have had pelvic surgery all have some damage to the sphincter (the valve at the opening of the urethra that regulates the flow of urine). Also, as we age, the spongy tissue around the sphincter shrinks, so it does not close as tightly. Our pubococcygeus (pelvic floor) muscles lose their zap, too, so we are unable to squeeze tightly to stop the urine. Really embarrassing, but not terminal. There are some things you can do. For starters, practice your Kegel exercises (see page 167) every chance you get, ten times a day at least. It's amazing how quickly you can strengthen those muscles and start to regain control.

A word of warning: do not get into the habit of piddling every time you are near a john. If you do, your bladder can shrink so that its capacity to retain urine diminishes. If this happens, you will have to go even more often. But please do not hold off till your back teeth are floating, with the idea that you will stretch your bladder and increase its capacity. You will, but so much so that the bladder will become atonic (overdistended) and lose its tone.

Now, there may come a day when no amount of Kegel exercises will help. If this happens, go to your doctor and ask for a referral to a urologist, who will do some tests and may recommend some new treatment. Hormone replacement therapy (estrogen and progesterone) may help postmenopausal women.

Under local injection, a specialist can inject a very small amount of collagen (a fatty, waxy substance) around the sphincter. This puffs it up and allows the sphincter to clamp shut and stop the flow of urine. This procedure lasts six to eight months and can be repeated. And it works.

Very occasionally, if a specialist finds scar tissue in the urethra and meatus (opening), surgery may be suggested. This requires a skilled surgeon. I would go for a second opinion.

If all else fails, well, today we have a new adult disposable diaper, and although it is bulky, it does the job. So this condition does not have to control your life and pleasure.

Males also often suffer incontinence, generally the symptom of an enlarged prostate gland. This may be the result of an infection (prostatitis) or a tumor or growth in the prostate gland.

Dear Sue: I've got a problem. I have trouble starting to urinate and find it impossible to stop once I get going. I dribble all the time, so I wrap a man-size Kleenex around my penis to keep from wetting my pants. Okay, so we expect this at seventy, but I am only thirty-eight. I hate to think what I will be like at seventy. I don't drink any fluids, but that does not help. I also have a heavy hot sensation down in my groin, and it ain't horny, believe me. Can you help?

Sue says: Absolutely. First make an appointment immediately with your doctor for a physical exam, including a prostate exam. (Take a sample of urine with you just in case.) Until you get your appointment, start doing Kegel exercises (see page 167) to increase your muscle tone and strength.

If your doctor diagnoses an infection of your prostate, he will give you a prescription for antibiotics to take for two weeks. Do take all of the pills, then go back to your doctor to make sure the infection has cleared up. It can become chronic and difficult to cure, so do as you are told. Do start drinking much more water. And if you are going to have sex, please use a condom to protect your partner because if there are bacteria in your urethra, it could infect her. Not nice.

Now, there is the remote possibility that you have an enlarged prostate from a growth or tumor. This can be diagnosed when your doctor does a rectal examination. Again, you will be referred to a urologist who will do tests and may recommend surgery. This would be unusual at your age, but at seventy, it is a possibility.

INFERTILITY

Dear Sue: *We have been married for three years. We used condoms and foam combined with the calendar method for the first year; then we decided we wanted to start a family. But* *so far, no luck at all. How soon can we start fertility testing and what is involved?*

Sue says: If you have been having unprotected sex on a regular basis for a period of one year without conception taking place, your family doctor may start testing in order to find out what is or is not happening. (She might refer you to a specialist or a "fertility clinic" for this testing.) Unfortunately, infertility is not uncommon. One in six couples experience infertility: 33 percent is caused by male factors and 33 percent by female factors, and the remainder is attributed to combined causes or is never explained. Infertility testing is covered by some medical insurance plans, but if you have to pay out of pocket, it can be very, very expensive.

The first appointment will involve a complete physical exam for the woman, with blood tests, urinalysis, and an in-depth personal and family medical history. The man will also get a physical exam and will have to provide a sperm sample, so that low sperm count or other problems can be ruled out (see page 171). Testing the male is relatively simple and treatment is usually effective, whereas the female causes are more varied and difficult to diagnose and treat. Female problems may include failure to ovulate regularly or at all, hormone imbalance, obstructions in the reproductive system resulting from pelvic inflammatory disease or endometriosis, antibodies to sperm in the cervical mucus, and structural or functional problems of the cervix or uterus.

Testing for the woman will begin with instructions for the couple to keep an accurate calendar that marks the onset and ending of the woman's menstrual period and notes every time they had intercourse and whether the man ejaculated. The woman must take her temperature every morning and chart it, in order to watch for the one-degree rise that indicates she is ovulating. She must also monitor her vaginal secretions at least twice a day.

After menstruation, a woman's vaginal secretions will be thick, heavy, and waxy, with a creamy color. They will remain that way about a week, give or take a few days. The secretions will then change and become thin, clear, and stringy (like uncooked egg white), indicating that she is about to ovulate. This will last about four days. Following ovulation, she will have "dry days" until her next period comes. Generally, a woman will ovulate fourteen days before her next period is due. To find out the length of her menstrual cycle and whether ovulation is occurring at the fourteen-day mark, you need a very accurate three-month menstrual chart.

Once ovulation has been confirmed, the doctor will ask the couple to make an appointment anytime from two to six days before the time she will be ovulating. The morning of that appointment, the couple has intercourse (she should avoid having a bath afterward). At the doctor's office or clinic, a sample of her cervical mucus will be collected and examined under a microscope to see if the sperm are alive and mobile. This will tell the doctor if her cervical mucus is hostile and killing off sperm. They may also do a biopsy of uterine lining to ensure that implantation can occur.

If the woman is ovulating, they will start to look for blockage of the fallopian tubes. They may order X-rays or an ultrasound. The doctor may order a hysterosalpingogram. Don't let the name scare you. *Hyster* means "uterus"; *salping* means "fallopian tubes"; and *ogram* means "X-rays." This test is performed after menstruation and before ovulation. A small tube is inserted into the cervical canal and a dye that can be seen with X-rays is slowly injected into the canal. The dye's passage through the uterus and into the fallopian tubes is monitored by a fluoroscope and by the X-rays that are being taken at the same time. If the fallopian tube is blocked, doctors may dilate and open the tube by inserting a flexible wire with a balloon on the end into the tube. The balloon will then be inflated and drawn out slowly, increasing the diameter of the opening in the tube. This test will probably be uncomfortable, so have somebody there to talk you through it and drive you home after. And don't panic: there will be a gooey discharge for some hours after. (Bring sanitary pads.)

If that was all clear, the doctor will probably do a laparoscopy. No panic: *lapar* means "going in through the abdominal wall"; *oscopy* refers to an instrument that is used to see things. (Before you are through with these tests, you will be able to rattle off these medicalese terms like the true "pro" that you will be.) Laparoscopy may be done to locate ovarian cysts and fibroids, endometriosis, and to find ova, or eggs, that are due to ripen and be released.

After giving the patient a general anesthetic, the doctor will make a tiny incision in the abdomen and will insert the laparascope. The laparascope consists of a light, fiber-optic lens and retractable surgical instruments and allows the surgeon to look at the reproductive organs. While you are under anesthetic, the doctors may also do a hysteroscopy, in which they insert a scope through the cervix and visually examine the uterine cavity.

These tests may reveal all is normal, but show that the woman may not be ovulating. She may then be placed on medication to induce ovulation. One of a number of drugs may be prescribed if hormone levels are normal, but the brain is not giving the pituitary gland the signal to release the hormone necessary for ovulation. She starts taking these pills on the fifth day after menstruation starts and continues taking them for five days. She may experience hot flashes, drowsiness, abdominal pain, breast tenderness, headache, dizziness, nausea, vomiting, and fatigue. Other drugs are used if the patient is deficient in hormones; they will help the eggs ripen. When the eggs are ready, an injection of a hormone that triggers ovulation is given.

Ovulation usually occurs five to eight days after the woman has taken her last pill. The couple should then have intercourse at least every other day beginning the third day after the last pill. Sounds like fun, eh? They can repeat this process for six months; then they should stop so that any possible negative side effects from the drugs may be avoided.

We are not through yet. If the woman is ovulating normally, but something is preventing conception and implantation, then the fertility specialist can give drugs that trigger ovulation of more than one egg. These drugs are often given in conjunction with artificial insemination. If this procedure is unsuccessful, a couple must decide whether they are willing to move into the "high-tech" realm of infertility treatment. If so, the doctor may proceed with an in vitro fertilization process. The woman will be given drugs to trigger multiple ovulation, and just prior to ovulation, a laparoscope will be used to retrieve those eggs and fertilize them in the lab. Fertilization will take place with sperm (the partner's if available or a donor's sperm if necessary and requested) that has been washed and centrifuged to concentrate it. A small tube is inserted into the woman's uterus and the fertilized egg (or eggs) is deposited, in the hope that one or more eggs will implant successfully.

There is also a new procedure called GIFT: Gamete Intra-Fallopian Transfer. Basically, ovulation is stimulated by the use of drugs. Ripened eggs are then retrieved and sperm obtained from the male partner. The sperm is washed, centrifuged, and put in a catheter (a long, hollow, soft plastic tub with a rounded, sealed end and a few openings toward the tip) along with the eggs. This mixture is then injected into the fibrillated ends of the female partner's fallopian tubes. Here, fertilization occurs naturally and the resulting embryos move down toward the uterus for implantation.

I make it sound so simple, but sorry, it isn't.

- It is very expensive.
- There can be negative side effects from the medications.
- The procedures are time-consuming and cause discomfort. They may also cause infection and bleeding.
- Other risks include multiple pregnancies, ectopic pregnancy, and miscarriages.
- It can take a long time.
- Infertility can take a toll on the relationship. The woman may become depressed if the treatment is not successful and she has a period or miscarries.

Do insist on accurate statistics of the success rates of your doctor or clinic before you decide on whether a procedure is for you. Remember to ask for the number of women who actually delivered a live, full-term baby, not the number of women who got pregnant (and may or may not have lost the pregnancy or who did not carry the baby full-term). Be very selective in your choice of clinics.

And don't overlook the enormous emotional strain fertility and infertility treatment places on both of you. Once a couple realizes that it is just not happening for them, they go through an almost predictable pattern of grieving, similar to grieving experienced with death and dying. In the beginning there is shock and surprise. Then there is denial: "This is not happening to us!"

The couple often feels alone and is unwilling to talk about their difficulties with family and friends. They may be embarrassed and feel that there is something "wrong" with them. They might find themselves avoiding family gatherings so they don't have to answer questions about when they will start a family. And seeing children may cause pain instead of pleasure: other people's children are a reminder of loss and fear that "it may never happen for us."

To these feelings of sadness, despair (even desperation), loss, and mourning, add guilt. Couples may feel they are being punished for past sexual activities with others or may wonder if she stayed on the Pill too long. And of course, a couple may also experience real anger over the situation: she may be mad that she used birth control for so long and that she has put up with the discomfort and inconvenience of menstruation for all those years for nothing. They may both be angry that they waited so long to try to get pregnant. (Fertility does decline somewhat during the thirties and dramatically in the forties, although women may remain fertile into their fifties.) The stress of infertility can affect men and women quite differently. It is often tougher for women because society generally assumes it is her "fault." Most of the testing and treatment tends to focus on the female. And every time she gets her period, she is reminded of failure and is devastated.

Men have their own problems. Now there is real pressure to "perform on command" whenever she thinks she is ovulating; at other times he has to cut back on intercourse to maintain a high sperm count. Sex loses its love, spontaneity, and fun. Instead it becomes a chore: a dirty job, but somebody's gotta do it.

Are there alternatives? Some women have claimed that going on a macrobiotic diet for six months set them straight.

Stress is a factor in infertility; don't let the stress of wanting a baby and wanting one now get in the way of conception. It's not uncommon for a couple to try, try, and try for a pregnancy, and when they get to the "end" of their options, they decide to adopt. Or they decide to be happy as a twosome. And lo and behold, nine months later, they've got a child.

The final emotion in the pattern should be "resolution." If nothing is successful, you may benefit from counseling to help you work through your feelings. You and your partner may decide to call it quits and consider living "child-free," or you may want to consider adoption. But getting to that decision is not easy, as the next letter tells us.

Dear Sue: *We were not able to get pregnant and ran the whole gamut of tests and treatment. The end result was no baby, no sex, no relationship. Everything else got put on hold while we devoted our lives to getting pregnant. The only thing we talked about was "the baby"; sex was "to make a baby." My wife wouldn't go for a bike ride because it might trigger a miscarriage, wouldn't have a drink because she might be pregnant. We spent so much money on treatment that if we had had a baby, we could not have afforded it. Now she is depressed and feels worthless and says I should find a wife who can give me the son she thinks I want. All I want is our life back.*

Sue says: Fast. Find a good marriage and family therapist and make an emergency appointment to give you something to hold on to and work toward. Also, make an appointment with your family doctor to see about her depression.

Together you are going to have to restructure your life and move away from thinking about menstrual cycles and the next doctor's appointment. Try to find a support group in your area. You can contact RESOLVE: The National Infertility

Association, 1310 Broadway, Somerville, MA 02144; phone 888-623-0744; www.resolve.org; to find out if there is a group in your area. You might also contact the Infertility Awareness Association of Canada, 2100 Marlowe Ave., Suite 39, Montreal, Quebec H4A 3L5; phone 514-484-2891; fax 514-484-0454; www.iaac.ca.

And start reading some of the books listed below: *Ended Beginnings: Healing Childbearing Losses* by Claudia Panuthos and Catherine Romero (New York: Warner, 1987); *In Pursuit of Fertility* by Robert R. Franklin and Dorothy Brockman (New York: Henry Holt, 1990); *The Gynecological Sourcebook* by M. Sara Rosenthal (New York: McGraw-Hill, 2003), 4th ed.; *Taking Charge of Your Fertility* by Toni Weschler (New York: Quill, 2001), rev. ed.

INTERNET PORNOGRAPHY

Dear Sue: *My thirteen-year-old son is spending a lot of time on the computer, and whenever we come by he quickly moves to another screen. Should I be suspicious?*

Sue says: Although there are a few women who enjoy hard-core pornography, most women regard it as degrading and threatening to their relationship. Most women do not have the sexy body seen in *Debbie Does Dallas*, nor are they willing to perform all the sex acts Debbie does. Some women believe their partner prefers masturbating to porn over having sex with them.

Porn can be destructive to a relationship; when talking about it seems to go nowhere, the anger and resentment build. And because women often feel powerless to stop their partner, many refuse to have sex with them, or if they do have sex, they may be seething inside.

Most couples have found that counseling with a good sex therapist is the only solution to the porn problem.

INTERNET SEX

Dear Sue: *I suspect my wife is having an affair with someone on the Internet. How does this work?*

Sue says: We used to believe that only males were involved in "chat rooms" and talking dirty on the internet, but it has become obvious that women also find it to be a very pleasurable pastime.

Problems arise when the one partner discovers that the other has been fooling around on the "net." They regard it as unfaithful that their trusted beloved is chatting up and sharing intimacies (and more) on the Internet.

Generally, the chat room conversation is innocent, but usually leads to talking dirty and describing sexually arousing scenarios. To obtain sexual release, one or both masturbate, complete with moaning and groaning.

Once again, this behavior will not be appreciated by the other partner, and may lead to destructive arguments and threats of divorce.

Before you go that route, please make an appointment with a good sex therapist for counseling. Therapy may seem a little expensive, but when you consider the emotional and financial costs of divorce, it is a good investment.

[j]

JEALOUSY

Dear Sue: *My girlfriend is so jealous. She gets mad if I even talk to another female. At a party, she created a really embarrassing scene when I spoke to another woman, and then she stormed home and wouldn't speak to me for a few days. She admitted she overreacted, but at another party she did it again.*

Sue says: Jealousy is an expression of fear and the need to control. She is feeling threatened, vulnerable, and powerless. It is painful and makes her crazy to the point that she goes off the deep end. She's irrational till she gets home and "chills out." Rather than identify what triggers this jealousy, she tries to eliminate the cause by controlling your behavior.

Jealousy is possessiveness. She wants you exclusively. Her self-concept and self-esteem may be wobbly, so she needs constant reassurance that you belong to her. What she does not realize is that you can never possess anybody. You cannot own another person. Nor can you control a person to the extent that they must not have contact with anybody of the opposite sex. That eliminates 51 percent of the world's population.

If she does not move beyond this need to control, your resentment will accumulate and you will become angry and rebellious. From there, your feelings toward her will begin to change. You will likely begin faultfinding to balance the power in your relationship. Ongoing criticism is damaging and will eventually destroy the love.

Obviously, talking and reasoning with her is not having an effect. However, you must be sure that you are not simply "pushing her buttons," and that you are not deliberately doing things to irritate her. This would give you power and control in the relationship.

You would both benefit from conjoint counseling. A therapist can help you learn new communication and listening skills. Your girlfriend will need to examine her own insecurity. What has happened in the past that makes her so jealous? Once you are both aware of what is happening, you can move toward increasing the trust level and helping her to develop her autonomy, independence, and sense of herself as a valuable person.

A therapist can help her develop different and more effective skills for coping with her feelings rather than running away and pouting for days. As soon as your partner feels capable and competent, she will not need to control you. When she is not playing the heavy, she will be more fun to be with, so you can both mix and mingle, and you will be back for the last dance.

I recommend an old but good book by Nancy Friday, *Jealousy* (New York: Bantam Books, 1991).

[k]

KEGEL EXERCISES

Dear Sue: *My husband feels that my vagina became too sloppy after the kids were born. I went to the gynecologist to see if they could snug it up a bit, and the doctor said no, but told me to do Kegel exercises. I have phoned my department of health, the La Leche League, looked at* Our Bodies, Ourselves, *and can only find a few vague lines on them, no instructions. Do you know where I can get them?*

Sue says: You came to the right place. Yes, Kegel instructions are hard to find. Mine came from the Ontario Midwifery Association. They are beneficial for men, too, and will help them maintain urinary control and as therapy for premature ejaculation.

We have a set of pubococcygeus (pelvic floor) muscles that support our lower abdominal organs. After rapid weight gain, pregnancy, or lower-abdominal surgery, they do get sloppy. You may also inherit a tendency to poor muscle tone. No excuse, exercise helps.

There is also another set of muscles called sphincters that clamp down and close off the urethra and the rectum, and there are a few of these around the vagina. All these muscles lose tone with pregnancy, surgery, and age.

As women and men age, they should practice Kegels after surgery, bladder infections, and weight loss. Women should also do them during pregnancy and after delivering a baby. You can reduce the possibility of urinary or stress incontinence (see page 153), tighten up the vagina, and increase your sexual pleasure. Women who have strong pubococcygeus muscles are more successful at reaching G-spot orgasm. Males will be able to "last longer" and enjoy sex more.

Now for the exercises—no membership at an exclusive fitness club is needed. First, you sit on the john (men, too), and start to urinate. Halfway through, try to stop and shut off the flow of urine without squeezing your legs together. If you can't do that, you should start the exercises now. Every time you go to the bathroom, try to do this start-stop repeatedly. This is called the "faucet." You will be amazed, because in about two weeks, you start to regain control. You're not through yet. Make it a habit—every time you urinate, stop-start to maintain sphincter control.

The "wave" can be done in the car when you are stuck in traffic or at a stoplight, while you are doing the dishes, working at your desk, or watching TV. Slowly tighten all the pubococcygeus muscles and sphincters. Feel your genitals pull up and in. Fantastic. Now hold for a count of ten, then slowly release. Do this ten times in a row, ten times a day.

Although it is not a Kegel exercise, if you are doing abdominal exercises—you know, the "crunches" where you lie on your back, bend your knees with your hands behind your head, and then raise head and shoulders up—for an added twist, make a conscious effort to tighten up your PC muscles. Two for the price of one.

Another fun one. Lying on your back, keep your knees apart and bent, your head and shoulders on the floor, and raise your hips. Now flop your knees together and apart. When your hips are up, squeeze your genitals together; when your hips are down, relax.

You and your partner can do these exercises together—ya never know what could happen.

And when you are having intercourse, just for the fun of it, clamp down and grip his penis. Then release. Do this for your pleasure and for his.

Do read *The Forgotten Key: An Update on Kegel Exercises*, by Gail Riegeris (www.isofem.org).

[1]

LOW SEX DRIVE

Dear Sue: *Tell me we are normal. We have been married for four years. In the beginning we had sex daily, then weekly, and now we remind ourselves that we have not done it for a month. He says he is fine and I know I am fine. But I listen to others and they seem to be doing it at least once a day.*

Sue says: This is normal for you. Do not worry about what others are doing. Sex drive is like appetite: some love to eat; for others eating is not number one on their list of priorities. So it is with sex. Nobody believed that couple who phoned in to *The Sunday Night Sex Show* and claimed they had sex twenty-one times a day. Now, there are only twenty-four hours a day, so that is almost once an hour. Get a life.

Don't compare yourselves to others. As long as you are both satisfied and happy, you are normal. Our sex drive continually evolves as our life changes; the dynamics of our life and our relationship all affect the ebb and flow of our sexual desire and arousal. "If it ain't broke, don't fix it," as long as you are happy with your life.

Low sex drive is covered extensively in many books, including *Going the Distance: Finding and Keeping Lifelong Love* by Lonnie Barbach and David L. Geisinger (New York: Plume, 1993), *Hot Sex: How to Do It* by Tracey Cox (New York: Bantam, 1999), and *Pure Sex* by Ann Hooper (Boston: Thorsons, 2003).

LOW SPERM COUNT

Dear Sue: My husband has only one testicle. Will we still be able to have a baby?

Sue says: For a male, being potent is seen as an essential aspect of his masculine identity. When a woman experiences difficulty getting pregnant and there is no evidence that she is infertile, one of the first tests for male infertility is a sperm count.

To do a sperm count, fresh ejaculate is required. So, armed with *Playboy* magazine, a male will be left in a little room in the clinic to masturbate and ejaculate into a test tube. The ejaculate is examined immediately under a microscope, not only to count the number of sperm but also to check the sperm's motility and to see whether it is abnormal (two heads or two tails).

Males are considered infertile if they have fewer than sixty million sperm in every ejaculation. While only one sperm is required for conception, you need twenty million sperm per milliliter of ejaculate to fertilize one ovum. Sounds like overkill, but as the lead sperm swim through the vagina to the uterus, they die off and neutralize the inhospitable vaginal and uterine secretions. Then the next phalanx of sperm moves forward to neutralize the inhospitable secretions, and the last few sperm meet the egg, at which point conception may occur.

Sperm are produced in the testicles. For maximum production of sperm, the testicles must be five degrees cooler than the rest of the body. If a man has a low sperm count, there are several things he can do: wear loose floppy boxer shorts rather than jockey shorts; avoid long hot tubs and saunas; engage in moderate physical exercise and cut out smoking.

Infertility may be caused by a sexually transmitted disease, which can leave scar tissue blocking the vas (the little tube that leads from the testicles to the urethra).

If a woman wants to get pregnant and her partner has a low sperm count, the doctor would likely recommend that they abstain from sex until she is ovulating, which would give her a better chance of conceiving. Also, for males with low sperm count, fertility clinics are now prescribing Clomid, a drug that increases sperm count.

[m]

MASTURBATION

Most males have a pretty good idea about masturbation. They call it "glad-handing." They know it is normal, that they will not go blind or reduce their sperm count—when they get married, they will not be "shooting blanks." They also realize they will not become homosexual as a result of masturbation. (If this were the case, 98 percent of males would be gay.) Many young women have the idea that "nice girls" don't touch their own genitals, but by the time women are in their early twenties, many give themselves permission to learn about their own sexual responses by solitary masturbation.

However, here is a common question from males.

Dear Sue: *I know how guys masturbate, but I just cannot imagine how females do it. They don't have a penis.*

Sue says: Because men focus only on stimulating their penis, they are at a loss to imagine how women (who must be anatomically deprived!) can possibly pleasure themselves. Most females reach orgasm by clitoral stimulation, not by vaginal stimulation. This explains why many use a vibrator to stimulate their genitals, rather than using it to mimic the thrusting of intercourse. Males have two basic masturbatory patterns: manual stimulation to ejaculation, or lying on top of a pillow and rocking. They call it humping the pillow.

Compared to men, women are very innovative. Many use manual stimulation, touching and stroking their genitals, or they may use a portable showerhead. (Don't just turn on the shower, let the shower turn you on.) She will lie in the bath in warm water, her legs up on the wall, allowing warm water from the tap to flow over her genitals. A woman may plan a romantic evening for herself with candlelight, a glass of wine, mellow music. Some women straddle the arm of the sofa and rock, and others have developed a technique of flipping into a favorite fantasy, and simply squeezing their legs together and squirming, even on the bus.

Unfortunately, too many women are still caught up in the idea that masturbation is morally wrong, especially for females. They believe "nice" girls do not pleasure themselves. Actually, sex therapists give anorgasmic women (females who have never reached orgasm) permission to masturbate and instructions for how to do it. When they learn how to bring themselves to orgasm, they can share that information with their partner, incorporating the different moves into their lovemaking. For a woman, masturbation is sexually liberating.

Dear Sue: *I can bring myself to orgasm very easily but can't reach the peak when we have sex.*

Sue says: Not uncommon. In solitary masturbation, you can do exactly what you want, how you want, when and where you want it. You do not have to worry about how you look, how you smell, how you sound, or whether your partner is getting bored or frustrated. You only have to worry about yourself, so it works. Masters and Johnson came to the conclusion that the level of sexual arousal and the orgasm is higher with solitary masturbation than when you have sex with your partner. This applied to both men and women. So is it any wonder people really enjoy pleasuring themselves?

Now we gotta be honest here—you are missing out on the body contact, the hugging, touching, kissing, the words of love and adoration, and that wonderful sense of bonding and togetherness, of being one with your partner. That is why sex with a beloved partner ranks high on our list of favorite pastimes. The excitement and thrill of sex with a new partner is also hard to beat.

Can you talk to your partner the next time you are having sex and very gently guide him to do what you like? Take his hand and place it where you want to be stroked and guide him as to the pressure and speed you prefer. If you like oral-genital sex, put his head where you want it. You know what works for you. Men don't know by divine intuition exactly what you want, so it is up to you to guide your lover.

That may be embarrassing. You may feel a little sleazy, but in reality you are taking the guesswork out of sex and taking the performance pressure off him. He will appreciate your talents.

Nowhere is it written that you cannot pleasure yourself during intercourse. He may find it awkward to stimulate your clitoris, so hey, you have a free hand, why not do it yourself? He won't mind, and you won't either.

Dear Sue: *Is it okay to use vegetables to masturbate?*

Sue says: Absolutely, providing you wash the carrot, zucchini, or cucumber first. Do be gentle because you can develop small painless tears in the mucous membrane. Risky if you have intercourse with a partner who is HIV positive without using a condom, which would be foolish in any case.

It is unfortunate that our society has placed so many negative injunctions on masturbation. It is safe, pleasurable, and harmless, and is used as one form of sex therapy for people with sexual dysfunctions.

For more information on female masturbation, read *The Magic of Sex* by Miriam Stoppard (New York: Penguin, 2001); *The Gynecological Sourcebook* by M. Sara Rosenthal (New York: McGraw-Hill, 2003), 4th ed.; *For Women Only: A Revolutionary Guide to Reclaiming Your Sex Life* by Jennifer Berman, M.D., and Laura Berman, Ph.D., with Elisabeth Bumiller (New York: Owl, 2002); *The Big Book of Masturbation* by Martha Cornog (San Francisco: Down There Press, 2003); and *First Person Singular* by Joani Blank (San Francisco: Down There Press, 1996). A great book for anorgasmic females is *For Yourselves* by Dr. Lonnie Barbach (New York: Signet, 1975).

MEETING "SOMEONE"

Dear Sue: *I have tried everything—dating services, companions wanted columns, the bar scene—with no luck. I am a reasonably good-looking guy and have a fair job. I meet a lady, have one date, and then get the kiss-off, "Can't we just be friends?" What am I doing wrong?*

Sue says: You may not be doing anything wrong. You just may not be the right person for that lady. Timing is important.

She may like you but not want to be in a relationship. Perhaps she is just coming out of a bad partnership and is not ready for the intensity that you convey. Better she should let you know now than date and delay till you are deeply involved and she bails out with a "Dear John" letter.

Could it be that you are selecting women who are impossibly glamorous, or fiercely independent? Right out of your league? (Am I being a snob? No. I go into schools and I am so aware of group distinctions—preppie, grunge, greaser, browner.) Whether or not it is a good thing, most kids are very selective and do not socialize out of their own stratum or league. Adults are very much the same. Do you have totally unrealistic expectations of what you want in a partner—someone who is intelligent, a high achiever, entertaining, and will make you look good?

Is your desperation palpable? Are you needy? This would scare her off. She may sense that you will become totally dependent on her for everything and contribute little or nothing to the relationship. Does she feel so smothered by your neediness that she makes a hasty exit?

Perhaps it is just bad luck, so try a new tack. Take up a new sport or hobby, a computer or gourmet cooking course, or auto mechanics for beginners. Go for coffee after. Slow and easy. Practice communication and listening skills. They come in handy.

MENOPAUSE, FEMALE

Until recently, "menopause" was an unmentionable word. However, now there is no shortage of information on the subject. Besides the availability of a number of good books, there are menopause clinics associated with most hospitals, as well as individual counseling and support groups. Today, most doctors are knowledgeable and willing to do more than pat you on the head and tell you it is normal and you will get over the "change of life." Unfortunately, they may simply prescribe hormone replacement therapy (HRT) without allowing you to make an informed choice. But you are not stupid and are quite capable of obtaining the information and deciding what is best for you.

Studies show that one third of women go through menopause with no problems, one third experience mild inconvenience and discomfort—hot flashes, night sweats—but are able to cope. The remaining third suffer severe osteoporosis (see page 198), insomnia, depression and/or mood swings.

Starting as early as age thirty, many women experience "perimenopause," a precursor to menopause with symptoms ranging from mood swings and irregular periods to hot flashes and vaginal dryness. Your doctor may prescribe the birth-control pill to make the transition easier.

Many women suspect that they may be going through menopause but are too embarrassed to find out for sure, or some just do not want to know. Some regard it as the time in life when one becomes an instant old lady, and others insist that it is simply *not* going to happen to them. As this letter shows, others just don't know anything about it.

Dear Sue: *My husband calls me "dingbat" à la Archie Bunker. My kids call me a flaky lady. I was a nice, normal, sedate fifty-one-year-old suburban wife with three teenage children. But all of a sudden, I am off balance most of the time and I feel old. What is going on here?*

Sue says: I don't like snap diagnoses, but it sounds like menopause to me. Most family doctors ask you to describe your symptoms. Hot flashes are a pretty good indicator, as are changes in your sleeping patterns and fluctuating moods from mad to glad to sad. Menstruation becomes irregular and gradually stops. Doctors confirm menopause when you have not had a period for at least one year. Until then, you must use some form of birth control or you could possibly have a "change-of-life baby."

There are other symptoms that you may be reluctant to discuss with your doctor. Your genitals become pale, dry, and lose their plumpness. Your vaginal walls become dry and thin without that spongy tissue behind, with less lubrication, so intercourse can be very uncomfortable. The walls of the vagina may crack or tear during sex, causing more pain and leaving you vulnerable to infections and cystitis. Not fun.

Please do not delay discussing such problems with your doctor. There is a simple estrogen hormone cream that can improve dry tissues very quickly. Hormone replacement therapy, which consists of estrogen and progesterone, may also be beneficial. HRT may be prescribed in the form of pills or a patch that adheres to the skin of your upper arm, abdomen, or hip. If you have had a hysterectomy, you do not need progesterone. If you are on HRT, you will have a light period every month. Ask your doctor about it, but then *you* make the choice. Another thing doctors do not tell you is that the more you have sex, the healthier your genitals will be.

Along with symptoms of menopause, women experience such signs of aging as redistribution of body fat, sagging breasts and floppy tissue under the arms and upper thighs, liver spots (age spots) on your skin, wrinkles, and gray hair. Fighting menopause is like trying to rearrange the deck chairs on the *Titanic,* although for some women hormone replacement therapy reduces the angst. Although there may be a slightly increased risk of breast cancer, this is offset by a dramatic reduction in lung cancer and osteoporosis. Read *Estrogen* by Nachtigal & Heilman (New York: Harper Perennial, 1994).

Here are some of the books about menopause that have flooded the market: *Menopause: The Complete Guide to Maintaining Health and Well-Being and Managing Your Life* by Dr. Miriam Stoppard (New York: DK Publishing, 2002), 2nd ed.; *Understanding Menopause* by Janine O'Leary Cobb (New York: Plume, 1993), rev. ed, is wonderful; *Is It Hot in Here or Is It Me? Facts, Fallacies and Feelings about Menopause* by Gayle Sand (New York: HarperCollins, 1993); *The Silent Passage: Menopause* by Gail Sheehy (New York: Pocket Books, 1998), rev. ed.; and *Before the Change: Taking Charge of Your Perimenopause* by Ann Louise Gittleman (San Francisco: HarperSanFrancisco, 1999).

MENOPAUSE, MALE (ANDROPAUSE)

Dear Sue: I am so weird I am scaring myself. Life has been good. I'm a fifty-six-year-old man, still married, and have four grandchildren. But I feel off balance. I am moody, have a low flash point, and am not even interested in sex. What the hell is going on?

Sue says: There are stacks of books written to help women through menopause, but you never even hear about a form of change of life that may affect men. And for many men, it is very real. Anytime after age fifty, a male's level of testosterone (the male sex hormone) fluctuates and gradually drops. Some doctors call it andropause. Any of these changes may occur in a man's life at this time:

- Mood swings, erratic and unpredictable moods not related to reality.
- Depression and a sense of failure because his career is not as successful as he had planned.
- Boredom with sex and thoughts like, "Is that all there is?"
- He may experience erectile failure with his partner but be attracted to a stunning young female. He may be tempted to try to woo and win her. If he does, he will be able to perform magnificently with her for six months, and then he will lose it again and be tempted to move on to find another partner.
- Dislike of the changes that are happening to his body—gray hair, wrinkles, and loss of muscle tone.
- Loneliness as the children become adults and leave home, accompanied by a feeling of being trapped or locked in and feeling that "the end is near."
- Resentment at getting older, frantically fighting normal aging.
- In an attempt to stay young, some men exercise to extremes, diet, take vitamins and queen-bee pollen, or get a Porsche.

The changes are difficult to take, and unfortunately men do not usually talk to anyone about them. Little has been written on male climacteric. You probably feel alone and scared. Can you find someone to whom you can talk about what is happening?

Do have a physical exam to ensure that you are healthy. If sexual performance is a concern, find a sexual-dysfunction or andrology clinic, or a good sex therapist. Perhaps you and your partner, who is also likely confused by your behavior, could benefit from relationship counseling.

You might find a support group of men who meet and share their experiences, which could provide reassurance that you are okay, and that might help you accept the natural aging process. I also recommend that you read *The New Male Sexuality* by Bernie Zilbergeld, Ph.D. (New York: Bantam, 1999).

Please don't try to just ignore it. What you are experiencing is real, and the long-term effects can be quite damaging to your relationship, especially if your partner is going through menopause at the same time. That could be a recipe for disaster. If your dream is to go into the future happily together, then finding help to get through this is essential.

THE MIDDLE YEARS

Unfortunately, our society has bought into the belief that by age eighteen males have reached their peak of sexual performance and from there on it is downhill all the way till about age fifty, when they truly lose it. We also think that females are late bloomers and do not reach their sexual peak until they are in their late twenties. If you have bought into this myth, you have shortchanged yourself. If you believe it, it will become a self-fulfilling prophecy.

Dear Sue: *I am a healthy thirty-five-year-old male. I have a great relationship with my wife, but it takes more to turn me on, it takes longer, and I don't get that same rigid erection I used to. Sometimes I lose my erection and the sensations during ejaculation are not as powerful. There are times when I suddenly realize three weeks have gone by since we have had sex. What is happening to "old faithful" who used to be up all day and half the night?*

Sue says: What you describe is not unusual. The expectation that you will have an ever-ready penis and your partner will have an ever-receptive vagina is totally unrealistic. The grand passion of young love, when you just could not get enough, has settled—fortunately, or else you would both have expired from exhaustion by now. You are into compassionate love, warm, comfortable, and intimate, with occasional flashes of brilliance. The "urge to merge" decreases as we get older, but our need for love and hugging and cuddling, for intimacy and connectedness, remains and becomes stronger.

There is something important here. Have you talked about your concerns with your partner? Is she satisfied with the status quo, or is she worried that you don't find her attractive anymore, or that you have someone else on the side? Would she feel comfortable initiating sex? Would she feel comfortable if your response were less than enthusiastic? Would you feel that you had failed yet again? Or could you laugh about it, call her a horny old broad, and reassure her that your penis just does not stand at attention on command, but when it does you'll be sure to let her know immediately?

Could you say, "The lights are on, but there's nobody home. Let's fool around till they arrive." Then you could pleasure her, stimulate her manually and with oral-genital sex, and if you get an erection, wonderful, go for it. But if not, it is not the end of the world. You can continue to stimulate her and maybe bring her to orgasm in other ways.

Did you know that most women do not reach orgasm with sexual intercourse, penis-in-the-vagina? Most women reach orgasm with clitoral stimulation. The clitoris is located about an inch above the vaginal opening, just below the folds of the labia, or lips. This pea-size organ is loaded with nerve endings, as many nerves as there are in a whole penis, and we all know how sensitive and responsive a penis is. Is it any wonder that clitoral stimulation must be very gentle—no grinding, instead a featherlight touch, kisses, licks, and sucking. So if we are unable to have intercourse, it does not mean "game over." Rather, it means we focus on other forms of stimulation.

Knowing that, you can eliminate your performance anxiety. You don't have to worry about getting a firm erection, nor do you have to worry about *keeping* a firm erection and being able to delay ejaculation long enough to satisfy your partner. No matter what happens, you are capable of giving her pleasure. Now you and your partner can both relax and enjoy. When you do stop worrying, you may find that old faithful rears its head once again!

Before we discard the penis as an unnecessary appendage, let me quickly tell you that, of course, most women enjoy the sensation of an erect, throbbing penis in their vagina. It provides a sense of togetherness, containment, fullness, and connectedness.

Let's face it, women like to take the credit when their partner has a humongous erection—"I'm good, I'm *that* good." This may be true, and it is good for her ego, so just accept it.

Here are some books that may give you some help: *The New Male Sexuality* by Bernie Zilbergeld, Ph.D. (New York: Bantam, 1999), and *The Magic of Sex* by Miriam Stoppard (New York: Penguin, 2001).

MISCARRIAGE

Dear Sue: *My period was late and I thought something was different, so I had a pregnancy test, which was positive. Then*

I had a period from hell, the doctor did another pregnancy test, and it was negative. Was the first test wrong?

Sue says: There are a few other things I'd need to know to answer your question. Is your period normally regular? Were you having sex during that cycle and were you using any method of birth control? If there were two yeses and a no, then I'd guess you were pregnant. Tests done by a laboratory are seldom wrong—the blood test, Beta HCG, is never wrong.

Please know that it is estimated that one in three first pregnancies ends up as a spontaneous abortion, so your story is not unusual. Most women go on to have normal, healthy babies, no problem. But to have a miscarriage during your first pregnancy is disconcerting. There is the fear that you may never get it right, that you might become a "habitual aborter," that you did something wrong, that God is punishing you, especially if you have had a therapeutic abortion in the past. This shame and blame is unfounded crap, so dump it.

Think about this. Each sperm and each egg is made up of twenty-three chromosomes that unite to make forty-six, and if even one chromosome is not completely normal, it can increase the risk of miscarriage. Most errors in chromosome numbers or constitution are accidental. Occasionally inherited chromosome abnormality predisposes one to miscarriage.

Miscarriages may also be caused by a malformed uterus, by a cervix that does not close tightly enough, by scar tissue or fibroids inside the uterus, by any hormonal imbalance, by exposure to drugs, alcohol, or smoking, or exposure to chemicals at home or at work.

Such common infections as measles, herpes, or hepatitis can cause spontaneous abortions, as can a mother's medical condition, which might include diabetes, lupus, or epilepsy. The mother's immune system may be unable to protect the fetus from tissue rejection.

As if that isn't enough, in later term miscarriages, there is the possibility that the placenta overlapped the cervical canal, or that the placenta separated prematurely, making way for an infection. There could also have been a knot in the umbilical cord or the cord could have become wrapped around the fetus, cutting off its supply of food and oxygen from the placenta and mother.

Now you know why we call birth a miracle. In all probability, you will get pregnant again and have the baby you want.

Dear Sue: I just lost a baby at four months of pregnancy. How soon can I get pregnant again?

Sue says: This is not carved in stone, but most doctors will suggest that you abstain from sex for a month until the bleeding and discharge has stopped, your cervix is closed again, and your hormones are back on track. You have to have had at least one normal menstrual period and a medical checkup.

Because pregnancy places great demands on your body, and because you need time to grieve the loss of that last baby, most doctors recommend waiting six months. Getting pregnant right away will never replace the loss of the previous baby. You and your partner need to be together and refocus. Unfortunately, there is not much support in our society for women and men to grieve over this kind of loss. But you've experienced a real loss, and you both need to mourn before trying again.

You may be scared to try again because you fear getting hurt again. That is why it is so important to heal. Read these great books: *Miscarriage: Women Sharing from the Heart* by Marie Allen, Ph.D., and Shelly Marks, M.S. (New York: Wiley, 1993), and *Preventing Miscarriage: The Good News* by Jonathan Scher, M.D., and Carol Dix (New York: Perennial, 1991).

Dear Sue: *I am what the doctor politely calls a "habitual aborter." Isn't that nice? Is there anything they can do to increase my chances of carrying a pregnancy to term?*

Sue says: You have likely been referred to an obstetrician/gynecologist who will try to identify what is going wrong. The problem could be.

- Bifurcated uterus, which means there is a divider down the middle.
- Incompetent cervix—it does not close up, so the embryo may be expelled.
- Insufficient hormones or a hormone imbalance.
- Genetic abnormalities in yourself or your partner.
- Congenital abnormalities affecting the embryo.

However, there are a few things you can do. Follow a well-balanced diet and engage in moderate exercise unless there is a problem, in which case doctors may recommend bedrest. You know about the risks of smoking and drinking alcohol. You need regular checkups with your obstetrician, who may put you on medication to promote "uterine quietude." It's also possible for your doctor to freeze your cervix and simply run a purse-string suture around the opening and snug it up until it is time to deliver the baby.

I am concerned about how you are coping emotionally with repeated miscarriages. You need the love and support of your partner, your family, and your friends. Please do not hesitate to get grief counseling to help you cope with this trauma.

MORNING-AFTER PILL

Frantic phone call to *The Sunday Night Sex Show:*

Oh, Sue! *We are so scared. Last night my girlfriend and I had sex and the condom slipped off. Is there anything we can do?*

Sue says: Don't panic—there is a chance that your girlfriend could use the early contraceptive pill, also called the morning-after pill, which prevents a fertilized egg from implanting in the uterus. However, you must act immediately.

On Monday morning, first thing, phone your family doctor, health department, or Planned Parenthood and ask if they prescribe the morning-after pill. If so, make an appointment for that day. This part is essential because the medication must be taken within seventy-two hours (three days) after unprotected sex or it will not prevent implantation of the fertilized egg. It is 98 percent effective but may not work if taken beyond that deadline. The doctor or counselor will want to know the exact date your girlfriend's last menstrual period started in order to establish whether she was ovulating at the time of the slippage. Be honest with the doctor or counselor because after seventy-two hours, conception and implantation of the fertilized egg may already have taken place.

Your girlfriend will be instructed to take two pills at 8 A.M. (I always tell women to take a Gravol pill twenty minutes beforehand because they might feel barfy). That evening, she should take another Gravol and then take the last two morning-after pills twenty minutes later. She may feel a little grungy all day, but she will probably not get pregnant. She will have a period in ten days to two weeks. If it's later than that, she should go back to her doctor or clinic for a pregnancy test.

While she is waiting for her period, she must use a reliable method of birth control if you are going to have sex. The morning-after pill is *not* a method of birth control, so the two of you should get an effective method of birth control immediately in addition to using a condom. You do not need this kind of stress and hassle in your life.

[o]

OFFICE RELATIONSHIPS

Dear Sue: *I am married, and my husband and I are great together. I have an executive job and work very closely with a male colleague on many projects. We have become a real team; we think alike, solve problems easily, and have spontaneous flashes of brilliance. I am becoming aware that there is a bit of chemistry bubbling just below the surface. We have never acknowledged it to each other, but I am sure he feels the same way. I am able to go home and thoroughly enjoy my husband, but I wonder how he would feel if he knew how well my work partner and I relate to each other.*

Sue says: In the past, males used to have all the executive power, while females were "just" secretaries. In a modern, egalitarian office atmosphere, men and women share many things in common: they may have comparable educational and socioeconomic backgrounds and similar interests, attitudes, and values, plus mutual ambition and a new feeling of understanding and acceptance. They often enjoy challenging one another, bouncing ideas off one another, brainstorming, and being imaginative and innovative. Very exciting, very stimulating.

A sense of trust develops, and along with it a sense of intimacy. You feel you know this coworker, you can trust him, you like him. There is a possibility that you will share a glance, and all of a sudden you realize—POW—that was different.

Now you gotta get smart here. You need to realize that there can be energy and synergy between two people without sex—intimacy does not necessarily mean that sex follows. It would be best, if you were sure he feels the same way you do, if you could talk to your coworker about your feelings. Use statements like, "I am aware that my feelings about you have undergone a change. I like you and I find you very attractive [interesting], and I enjoy working with you." Honesty is the best policy, not denial, so you could say something like, "I must admit, these different feelings scare me because I am happily married. I love my husband dearly and do not want anything to jeopardize that relationship."

Here, you have used "I" terms, which makes it safer; you have left it open for your coworker to say how he/she is feeling, and have been very clear about what the bottom line is for you.

You have set clear boundaries for this relationship that is more than a friendship. This will *not* become a love affair; it will not become sexual, so there will be no physical contact and no "language of lovers." You both agree to respect each other's privacy and personal identity. You both must adhere to these boundaries.

Do not try to hide this working friendship from your partner. He knows that you work with both men and women; he understands mutual attraction and trusts your integrity and will not feel threatened. By talking about your situation at the office and being honest, your partner will know that you are not keeping secrets and that you are not feeling guilty because there is nothing to feel guilty about. The difference between the two situations is that you love your partner, while you enjoy the dynamic working relationship with your colleague.

If you are open with both your partner and your co-worker, the excitement, the productivity, the mutual admiration and respect can continue. Enjoy the chemistry of both relationships. The attraction can be shared and enjoyed and benefit you, your coworker, and your work, and there it stays.

Dear Sue: *I work in the personnel department of a large corporation. I am middle management, working with five others. The boss was a male whom I really liked. We started with working lunches, which moved into "a little afternoon delight." Not smart. The others on the team resented us taking time out and they were sarcastic and accused the boss of playing favorites. They implied that we were having sex in the supply room (we were caught kissing in there) and they complained to the top dog. They also claimed there was favoritism and that I got all the easy cases. The upshot was that I was fired, he was demoted, and we went through an ugly breakup. Please, tell folks not to get involved in an office romance. It is a bad scene.*

Sue says: This letter kinda tells it all if you allow an attraction to move into a sexual relationship in the workplace. But you are not powerless when in lust and love. You can call the shots and remain in control within the boundaries to which you have agreed.

ORAL SEX

As I said in my introduction to this book, I use two kinds of language: street slang, which is comfortable and familiar; or proper medical terminology, which is safe, inoffensive, and, to many, incomprehensible. The latter includes terms like "cunnilingus" (oral sex performed on a woman) and "fellatio" (oral sex performed on a man). I like to flip-flop between them. So when you read "blow job," "giving head," "going down on her," or "eating her out," do not be shocked. You cannot talk sex without being explicit, and sometimes explicit is graphic.

Dear Sue: *How can I give my boyfriend a blow job without feeling I want to barf all over him?*

Sue says: There is no right or wrong way to perform oral sex on a male, but it is a skill you can develop. You need to find out what he likes, what feels good for him. Then, when you take his penis into your mouth, drool—you need lots of saliva to provide lubrication. Do not go way down on the shaft. Instead, hold the base of his penis in hand, and coordinate your head and your hand rhythm together to stimulate the length of his penis. This is every bit as pleasurable for him and lets you avoid that feeling that you are going to flip your biscuits. With your free hand, stroke his testicles and the area around his anus. He will think he has died and gone to heaven. Ask him to tell you if he wants you to be gentle or firm, slow or fast, higher or lower on his penis. Only he knows what he would like.

Dear Sue: *Can you get AIDS from giving head?*

Sue says: Oral-genital sex is regarded as low-risk behavior for the transmission of the HIV virus, providing there are no breaks in the mucous membrane of the performer's mouth. That means, no herpes lesions, no cankers, no gumboils, no root-canal work done that day, no sores from chomping down on your lip or biting your tongue while eating a sub. These breaks in the mucous membrane of your mouth or lip could provide access for the virus if your partner is HIV positive and the virus is concentrated in his ejaculate. However, recent reports have suggested that the virus might also penetrate intact mucous membranes in the throat, so low risk doesn't mean no risk.

Now, if the performer, whether male or female, is HIV positive, a minute number of the virus will be concentrated in his/her saliva, but not enough to cause an infection, even if his/her partner has a gash on their genitals.

So oral-genital sex can be risky behavior for AIDS. There are other STIs that can be transmitted by oral sex. If either partner has herpes, either on the genitals or lips, they can infect the other partner. Or if one has a gonorrhea infection in the penis or vagina, that bacteria can get in the mouth and throat of the performer. Likewise, if the performer has pharyngeal (throat) gonorrhea, the recipient can be infected.

Dear Sue: *Why is oral sex so popular?*

Sue says: Because it feels good. It is sexually stimulating and exciting and is great as foreplay and as an alternative to sexual intercourse. You may be surprised to learn that sex therapists suggest oral sex as a form of therapy for many sexual dysfunctions, such as premature ejaculation, delayed or retarded ejaculation, and low sex drive in males and females. There are more good reasons:

- It reduces the risk of unplanned pregnancy.
- It can be performed by most people even if they have a heart condition or physical disability.
- Many people who are unable to reach orgasm with intercourse will be able to come with oral-genital sex.

Some of the myths about blow jobs are:

- Swallowing ejaculate will clear up your acne. Wrong.
- Swallowing ejaculate will give you big breasts. Wrong.
- Swallowing ejaculate will make you fat. Wrong. There are thirty-five calories in one teaspoon of ejaculate. And a male generally ejaculates only one teaspoonful each time.
- You can get pregnant swallowing ejaculate. Wrong.
- Swallowing ejaculate will eliminate menstrual cramps. Wrong. But reaching orgasm has been shown to help reduce cramps.
- Only gays perform oral sex. Wrong, all wrong.

Dear Sue: *My boyfriend loves it if I go down on him, but he will not do it for me. He thinks it smells bad.*

Sue says: Who told him that his genitals smell like a rosebud? Give me a break. Most women are more conscious of their genital odors than men are about theirs, so they have a bath regularly, and some even go to the extent of douching (not a great idea) and wearing deodorant tampons and sanitary napkins (again, not a great idea). Guys do not even wipe when they pee!

Now, he may be afraid that you have a sexually transmitted disease that he could get, or, there are some males who have a fear of the vagina. They believe it has teeth and can trap a male, chew him up, and spit him out! If these are his concerns about oral sex, how can he be comfortable putting his penis in your vagina?

Lady, you talk to him softly but firmly. Tell him if your vagina is good enough for his penis, his most precious part, then it should be good enough for his face. Another idea— why not wash each other as a sexy, soapy prelude to love-making?

Some women are not too comfortable allowing their partner to perform cunnilingus on them. They may be afraid he has an infection such as a cold sore (herpes). They may regard oral sex as abnormal. Perhaps a partner was too rough and they ended up with raw and painful genitals. There is always the possibility that oral sex triggers flashbacks of incest or sexual assault in the past. I would suggest that these people get good counseling to help overcome this trauma.

At the same time, many people simply like or dislike oral sex. These things are a personal choice.

ORGASM

Dear Sue: *I just can't seem to get there. I reach orgasm with masturbation by myself, but with my boyfriend, I get to a certain point and can't seem to get beyond that. I feel blocked.*

Sue says: Take a piece of paper and jot down all the "nice girls don't" messages that you got as a child. Injunctions like: "Don't sit with your legs apart." "Don't look at your genitals." "Don't kiss a guy on your first date." "Don't let him know you are horny." "For heaven's sake, don't forget to take a shower every day because your genitals don't smell very good."

Now, there you are, having wonderful "wet sex" with your boyfriend; your heels are up around your ears, and all those tapes are playing in your head. Suddenly you think, "He is going to think I'm a real slut. Hope he doesn't notice my thunder thighs. Yech, my genitals stink. He'll see the stretch marks and my breasts are under my armpit; oh, gross—"

You may also be thinking, "Gotta do it, gotta go over the top. He is going to think I'm frigid or that I don't love him or that I think he is a lousy lover. Gotta cum—why isn't it happening? Oh no, I'm losing it. That's it, game over."

You may also have the fear that you will simply lose control, flip out, look like some kind of crazed animal, or that he might think you are some kind of freak. So you keep a tight rein on yourself; you don't let go and just let it happen.

These preoccupations will distract you and prevent you from simply focusing on the pleasurable sensations of fondling, petting, oral-genital sex, and intercourse.

There is also the possibility that you have simply never guided your partner to do all the pleasurable, stimulating things that you do for yourself. Show him, tell him, lead him. He will love it, and I hope, so will you.

For more information about orgasm, please read some of these great books: *For Yourself: The Fulfillment of Female Sexuality* by Dr. Lonnie Barbach (New York: Signet, 2000), rev. ed.; *The Magic of Sex* by Miriam Stoppard (New York: Penguin, 2001); *Urge: Hot Secrets for Great Sex* by Dr. Gabrielle Morrissey (Thorsons, 2003); *Women's Sexual Passages: Finding Pleasure and Intimacy at Every Stage of Life* by Elizabeth Davis (Berkeley, Calif.: Hunter House, 2000); and *Great Sex Guide* by Anne Hooper (New York: DK Publishing, 1999).

Dear Sue: *I live in a frat house with a bunch of other guys, one of whom brings his girlfriend to his room for sex. Sue, she makes so much noise, moans, screams, yells "yes, yes, yes!" Is this normal?*

Sue says: We got the picture. This may be normal for her, or she may have been watching too many soap operas and is convinced this is the way it should be.

Call a residents' meeting, and as a group, tell your frat brother exactly how this behavior affects you. Perhaps you find it distracts you from your studies; perhaps you believe it is attention-getting behavior; perhaps it makes you horny; or perhaps it is embarrassing for everybody. These are all valid reactions to their inappropriate behavior—inappropriate in that setting.

Find out if this guy has any suggestions as to what he could do about it. He could either talk to the groaner and convince her this can't go on, or they could find another location. Gently but firmly set a deadline, say one month, and if at that point silence isn't golden, tell him he will have to find another place to live. She may simply be playing to a captive audience to make you all jealous and he may even be urging her on because it makes him look spectacular.

OSTEOPOROSIS

Dear Sue: *What is this osteo thing I keep hearing about?*

Sue says: I am so glad you asked about osteoporosis because it is serious but reversible with medication.

Your bones have calcium in them, and as you age, the calcium tends to come out, leaving bones brittle and porous. So if you stumble, you don't just twist your ankle, you break it. Somebody gives you a big hug and cracks a few of your ribs, or you notice you are shrinking and starting to become round-shouldered. Now, we cannot undo the damage that has already been done, but we can help prevent further damage. That's why it's important to get to your doctor as soon as possible. You can have a bone-density study to diagnose the condition of your bones.

Osteoporosis seems to affect females who have a fair complexion and blond hair, and are fairly slim. It tends to run in families and seldom affects women of color, dark-complexioned women, or heavy women. Generally, men are spared osteoporosis.

There are a few things you can do. Weight-bearing exercise increases absorption of calcium, so walking, low-impact aerobics (foot-to-ground exercises), light weight lifting, and cycling are all good. Eat a well-balanced diet that includes three to four glasses of milk a day, or another dairy product that will give you the equivalent calcium intake. Skim milk contains as much calcium as homogenized, so the fear of fat is no excuse. Research is also being done on fluoride supplements in relation to osteoporosis, so check that out. Ask your doctor about hormone replacement therapy to maintain bone density.

We are now hearing about a new medication called Fosamax that promotes calcium reabsorption to increase bone density, making porous bones stronger and reducing the risk of fractures.

Read the following books: *The Gynecological Sourcebook* by M. Sara Rosenthal (New York: McGraw-Hill, 2003), 4th ed.; *Dr. Susan Love's Hormone Book* by Susan M. Love, M.D., with Karen Lindsay (New York: Three Rivers, 1998); and *The*

Menopause Sourcebook by Gretchen Henkel (New York: McGraw-Hill, 2001), 3rd ed. These books will help you make an informed decision about hormone replacement therapy. It is safe and does not cause cancer. It is the only thing that works.

[p]

PAP SMEAR (INCLUDING OTHER DIAGNOSTIC PROCEDURES: COLPOSCOPY, CONE BIOPSY, CRYOTHERAPY)

Dear Sue: *I had a routine Pap smear last week, and the doctor phoned me to say the lab reports were "suspicious" and I was to come in for a repeat Pap. I am freaking out. Does this mean I have cancer?*

Sue says: Not to panic. They may want to repeat the test to be sure there are no mistakes or mixed-up reports, or to get a clearer sample. Let's get some bottom-line information here.

A Pap smear involves a swab to pick up cells and secretions from the cervix and top of the vagina. The doctor wipes the secretions on a glass slide, sprays it with a fixative, and sends it to a laboratory for examination under a microscope.

If abnormal cells are present, they will be seen, identified, and a report will be sent to the doctor.

A Pap smear will *not* diagnose such STIs as herpes, venereal warts (HPV, or human papilloma virus), or gonorrhea, but may indicate cell changes that occur if one of these STIs is present. Cells in the cervix change as a result of many factors, including sexual activity, aging, irritation, inflammation, or infection. A Pap smear indicates whether there are changes that should be monitored.

Each lab is different, but the report results may read "benign" (meaning all is normal, no problem) or "atypia benign" (indicating there are cell changes that should be monitored through a repeat Pap smear every six months—no cause for alarm). Some laboratories report "Stage 1," "Stage 2," or "Stage 3" and others, "mild," "moderate," or "severe" dysplasia.

At any stage, your doctor may order a *colposcopy.* No anesthetic is necessary for this procedure, which is done in the doctor's office with an instrument that incorporates a light and a microscope, allowing the extent of the cell changes in the cervix to be examined. The area will be stained with a mild solution of vinegar in water. The doctor may take a small biopsy at that time to identify cell changes that may be caused by HPV. If venereal warts are present, they will change color and be visible. Precancerous cells would show up at this time.

The next procedure is a *cone biopsy,* done under local anesthetic in the hospital. A small wedge, or cone, is removed from the bottom of the cervix. This is sent to the lab for microscopic examination, to confirm the extent and degree of the changes.

One doctor has a concise way to describe possible treatments: we can "freeze, heat, burn, or zap." In the procedure called *cryotherapy* (freeze), a flat metal probe is gently inserted into the cervical canal. It freezes and destroys abnormal lesions and cancers. This would be done in the gynecologist's office because no anesthetic is required. However, it does cause cramps, bleeding, and a stinky watery discharge for four to six weeks afterward.

In *loop diathermy* (heat), a thin wire loop that is heated with an electric current slices through the affected tissue and cauterizes (seals off by heat) blood vessels to reduce bleeding and hasten healing.

Electrocautery (burn) may be used if the problem area is not too extensive. The cancerous tissue or lesions are burned away with a metal probe through which an electric current passes.

In *laser treatment* (zap), a small beam of light hot enough to vaporize the cancerous tissues or lesions is focused on the cervix for about ten minutes. No anesthetic is required and there may be some bleeding afterward.

If the cancer is extensive, the gynecologist will suggest a hysterectomy. If there is a possibility that the cancer has metastasized (spread to other organs or the lymph nodes), radiation therapy will be suggested after surgery.

Prevention is essential. Venereal warts, almost an epidemic today, are an irritant to the cervix and may cause cancer in a small proportion of women. So if you are in a new relationship, or if you even suspect that your partner may not be faithful, then you must be responsible for your health and practice Safer Sex: insist on condoms.

All women must have a Pap smear every year. If you notice any small flat warts on your external genitals, go to a good doctor immediately.

Since Pap smears were made available to women in 1943, they have become a routine part of a woman's annual physical examination, and the death rate from cancer of the cervix has been reduced by 70 percent. All females aged eighteen or over, or from the time they start having sexual intercourse, should have an annual Pap. It's covered by most insurance and, if you don't have insurance, is a service offered for low cost at women's health clinics across the country. You have no excuse!

PENIS SIZE

Dear Sue: *Is bigger better? I am a twenty-two-year-old male who is hung like a hamster. I am embarrassed in the locker room, and I am terrified that a female will just crack up laughing if she sees my penis. Are there any exercises you can do, foods you can eat, creams you can rub on, vitamins you can take, or surgery you can have?*

Sue says: This is serious. Your anxiety is going to affect your whole life. You may settle for a lady who will not laugh instead of a lady you care about. So, in essence, much of your destiny is determined by how you feel about your small penis.

Let's look at some facts. The average nonerect penis is three and one half to five and one half inches long. When fully erect, it is five to seven inches long. Research tells us that the smallest nonerect penis is only slightly smaller when it is fully erect than the largest penis with a full erection. Believe it!

Penis size is inherited, and except in cases of congenital "micropenis," it is proportionate to the rest of the body.

Bigger is not better. In fact, too big can be a problem in that it could hurt your partner. It is what you do with what you've got that counts, no matter the size. That means genital petting and oral-genital sex to provide clitoral stimulation. You see, recent studies tell us that most females do not reach orgasm from a thrusting penis in the vagina. That is not where the best action is. The clitoris (that small round organ located just below the folds of the labia) is supersensitive and responsive to light touch, stroking, or licking. You do not need a large penis to do that. An active imagination is a real bonus, though. Do check with your partner to find out what moves are pleasurable for her.

The vagina is a tube, about four inches long; it is very elastic, lined with mucous membrane. The top two thirds of the vagina has very few nerve endings.

You don't believe me? Okay, ask any female who has ever worn a tampon. Once that tampon is inserted, she simply cannot feel it. If it weren't for the string, she might forget that it's in there. However, the lower one third of the vagina is loaded with nerve endings, wall-to-wall sensations. Now, the guy with the smallest penis is going to be in the bottom one third. What's the benefit of a ten-inch penis banging around in there when "there's nobody home"?

Also, you need to know that the walls of the vagina are elastic. They stretch enough to deliver a ten-pound baby, and the walls will not tear. So, unless the man has a ten-pound penis, a woman can take it. But she will need to be very aroused, lubricated, and relaxed.

Remember, too, that in intercourse you are both aware of the warmth, the throbbing sensations, the feeling of fullness and containment, and that sense of closeness, connected-ness, and bonding. That is a good feeling but does not lead to orgasm.

I would be less than honest if I did not tell you that for a woman, seeing her partner with a firm erection wanting *her*—wow—that is a real boost for her ego. She thinks, "He craves me. I am so good that I can get him that hot, let's go." Your attraction to her is the turn on, not the size of your pe nis. So carve that fact in stone, and be thankful you're not up against such problems as impotence, premature ejaculation, retarded ejaculation, or low sex drive.

Please believe me. If you can accept what I am saying, you will not need a penis "hard enough to drive a nail with or long enough to fly a flag from." There is absolutely no reason for performance anxiety and feelings of inadequacy because of penis size.

PEYRONNIE'S DISEASE

Dear Sue: *My sins of the past are catching up with me. I used to masturbate with my right hand. I knew this was wrong, and now I am being punished. My penis has a curve in it. Literally, it makes a right-angle turn. I am too embarrassed to have a shower after playing squash because all the guys will know what I did. And women will not even come near me with this angle of dangle. Is there anything I can do to straighten it out?*

Sue says: If what you say is true, then the cure would be so simple. All you'd have to do is to masturbate with your left hand and that would bring it around. But your problem, Peyronnie's disease, or chordee, is a fairly common condition among mature males. It has absolutely nothing to do with masturbation; otherwise most men would have a penis with a kink in it. (After you have read through this section, read the section on masturbation on page 173. It is essential to eliminate the guilt and shame that you are feeling about masturbation.)

Now for the medical explanation. Strands of dense fibrous tissue or heavy plaque develop in the spongy tissue of the penis, probably as a result of injury when you were a little guy. Perhaps you got hit playing hockey, fell off your bike and hit the crossbar, or were kneed in the crotch—painful, but you got over it. As you get older, the tissue shrinks and becomes harder on one side, pulling the penis in one direction. Some researchers have found an increase in fibrous tissue after a guy has been treated for an infection and inflammation called urethritis. Normally, with Peronnie's disease, your penis would hang okay and you would have no problem urinating, but with an erection it would deviate, sometimes quite dramatically.

This angle can make it difficult, if not impossible, for some males to have intercourse. Sex may be painful for them and uncomfortable or agony for her. Some males experience a slow or sluggish erection, which may be less rigid than it was before. The couple may avoid discussion out of embarrassment and try to pretend that everything is cool. They avoid all sexual contact—no hugging and cuddling, no petting, solitary or mutual masturbation, and no oral sex.

You need an appointment with your family doctor for a physical examination. You will probably be referred to a urologist (a specialist in urinary problems), who will also examine you and recommend treatment.

Peyronnie's disease has a tendency to get better on its own. The fibrous tissue may dissolve and be slowly absorbed without any treatment. That is fortunate, because there is no truly effective treatment. Researchers have tried vitamin-E creams and oral medication, hormones, including estrogen and other steroids, in an attempt to soften the tissue. Ultrasound and radiation therapy have also been tried. Some doctors recommend surgery to remove the tissue. In surgery, there is always the possibility that nerves will be damaged or that the blood supply to the penis will be disturbed, which could affect sexual performance. British urologists have found that shock-wave therapy can straighten a bent penis in men with Peyronnie's disease. A man needs three treatments, each a month apart, and some patients require more after six months.

Now that you have the facts about your curvature of the penis, I am concerned about the damage this has done to your self-concept and self-esteem. Because you blame yourself for what has happened and feel guilty about masturbation, you may feel that you are not worthy and that nobody will want you. Getting information and integrating the facts is one component. Now you need to learn to accept validation from others, and to validate yourself. Please make an appointment for sex counseling so you can work through your feelings of guilt and unworthiness.

You are a worthwhile person and you have a great deal to contribute to a relationship. When you feel good about yourself as a sexual human being, you can also feel you are a great lover in spite of a twisted penis! (You gotta laugh!)

A great start would be for you to read *The New Male Sexuality* by Bernie Zilbergeld, Ph.D. (New York: Bantam, 1999). You and your partner could both read *The Magic of Sex* by Miriam Stoppard (New York: Penguin, 2001).

PHONE SEX

Dear Sue: *The Visa bill came in the other day and there were these charges that really embarrassed my boyfriend. They were for phone sex, and I flipped out. We enjoy frequent sex together, so why the hell would he do this?*

Sue says: This is a relatively new phenomenon in the sex industry and is the ultimate in Safer Sex. Basically, you phone an advertised number and engage in very explicit dirty talk designed to trigger sexual fantasies. The person on the other end of the line will encourage you by saying things like, "O-o-oh, you are gorgeous! What a magnificent penis, bet you can make that bigger. What would you like to do with it? I am unbuttoning my blouse . . ." They will talk you through all the moves, making it last because you are being charged by the minute. They have to be good so that you will call again—soon.

If your boyfriend becomes addicted to phone sex, it will be expensive and he may need to seek counseling.

There are "love lines" for both men and women. Basically, they are harmless, and it does not mean that you are not a great lover because your partner is using them. It is something new, exciting, thrilling, and completely different. A woman on the phone will "talk dirty" to the caller to convince him she is hot for him. The caller does not realize that the woman is probably playing solitaire or knitting a sweater for her baby.

It might be beneficial if you wrote in a journal exactly how you feel about your boyfriend's pastime. Are you grossed out? Why? Do you feel inadequate or angry? Do you feel your relationship is threatened, or that he is "sick"? Be honest; this journal is just to help you focus on your feelings. You may decide it is not worth worrying about, or you may still be upset. You might also try reading *The Sexually Unusual: A Guide to Understanding and Helping* by Dennis M. Dailey (New York: Haworth Press, 1989).

Then you and your partner might be able to talk about it, and if you are unable to arrive at a satisfactory solution, you might need some relationship counseling. Please don't just ignore the problem, or assume it will resolve itself. Your resentment and suspicion will just get worse.

PIERCING

Dear Sue: *I want to do this for me, don't ask me why, but I want to have a ring put through my penis. Tell me what I need to know.*

Sue says: Body piercing ranges from earrings, nose rings, or studs, which you see every day, to those you don't see, unless you or your partner has body jewelry. Generally, a ring is about an inch across, as thick as the ring from a three-ring binder, not a closed circle but with a small knob at one end and a screw-on knob at the other. The studs are also called "bones," again with a bulge at one end and a screw-on bulge at the other that keeps it from falling out. Nipple rings or studs are very common for both males and females. Belly-button rings or studs are interesting, but what really grabs people are the genital rings or studs. Warning, don't read this if you are squeamish.

Males may have a "Prince Arthur ring" through the fore-skin or sometimes they will have it inserted through the urethra so that it exits just below and behind the head of the penis. Males tell me it does not hurt, but does increase their awareness of their sexual arousal. Some males leave it in during sex, but many remove it out of respect for their partner's comfort. It must be removed before a condom is rolled on.

Females may use beautiful studs with semiprecious jewels in the screw end, or they may have rings with jewels at the end. Now, you could use diamonds, but most commonly the rings are set with round smooth stones such as jade, opal, amethyst, amber, or red cornelian. Women may have one or many penetrating the labia majora (large lips of the female genitals). Some women add a new ring to celebrate special occasions—an anniversary, a new baby. Generally, these women shave off pubic hair so it does not get caught in the rings and tug. The women whom I know who have this jewelry regard it as private adornment. They are really proud of it and feel it enhances their sexuality.

Before you run out and have it done, there are a few things you gotta know. The piercing must be done by an experienced professional. This is not like going to Sears to get your ears pierced with an ice cube to numb the lobe. New, sterile instruments and gloves must be used and you must take time to find out exactly how to take care of the puncture to prevent infection. You need to be aware that if there is a tear or infection at the puncture site, and you have unprotected sex before it completely heals, you are at risk of getting HIV/AIDS. *No sex* for about four weeks after the piercing until it has healed and scar tissue has formed.

So this is not something you do one night on a dare, after too much to drink. Reputable operators insist on two appointments: one to tell you all about it and give you time to change your mind. If you still want one, you make an appointment to come back in a week. I must tell you that not everybody thinks body jewelry is "a thing of beauty and a joy forever." So if you are in a relationship, do discuss it with your partner so there are no little surprises when you come out flaunting a ring through your penis. If you have body piercing, do tell a new partner about it before you get into sex, and do use condoms, for the sake of both of you.

PILES (HEMORRHOIDS)

Dear Sue: The other day my girlfriend put her finger in my bum hole. The very next day, I developed a small pile, which bled a little bit when I went to the bathroom.

Sue says: The fact that your girlfriend penetrated your rectum with her finger would not cause piles or hemorrhoids. There are three major veins around the rectal sphincter, or opening, and one or more of these veins may prolapse or protrude outside the bowel if you were constipated and strained while having a bowel movement, or you had diarrhea and a vein was forced out; or, for women, during pregnancy, when the pressure of the baby and uterus may cause a vein to pop out. Sometimes the blood is still circulating in the vein; other times there is a thrombus, or clot, blocking the vein. Either way, the veins tingle, itch, burn, and throb.

Although what I have to suggest may not appeal to you, it will help. Wash your hands, put topical analgesic (Preparation H or Lanacaine) on your index finger, then around your rectum. And relax while you gently insert the vein(s) back into your rectum. Be sure to wash your hands again. You may need to do this several times a day and after each bowel movement until the hemorrhoids shrink.

If the bleeding is bright red, it means a small blood vessel is rupturing whenever you have a bowel movement. It will likely heal quickly. Old, dark blood means there is bleeding higher up in the bowel. This should be checked out by a physician. Homosexual males who frequently have vigorous anal sex are prone to hemorrhoids.

Do read the segment on anal sex on page 26 and the bottom line is, gently, Bentley . . .

POSITIONS

I have heard that there are at least 325 sexual positions. Now, if you are very agile, double-jointed, and flexible, you and your partner can experiment, using the old *Kamasutra* as a guide, and try to position yourselves as shown in those lovely drawings.

At worst, you will get stuck and someone will have to untangle you, or you might develop an agonizing cramp or spasm. At best, you'll have mind-blowing orgasms. The most likely scenario is that you both dissolve in "mirth quakes" and end up in the basic missionary position.

Dear Sue: *For a change of pace, my partner and I decided to expand our repertoire of sexual positions. We ran out of ideas. Can you give us some suggestions?*

Sue says: These are the most common, the most fun, and the most user-friendly.

Missionary: female on bottom, male on top. Then there's female superior, or female on top. Front to front, both lying on your sides, is less strenuous and good if there is a physical disability. An adaptation of that is great but difficult to describe: the man and woman lie side by side, both on their backs; she slides over him crosswise, like an *X;* they spread their legs so that they overlap as the bottom of the *X,* and his penis enters her vagina from behind. You still with me?

The old spoon position: they both lie on their sides, his front to her back, he enters her from behind.

Standing position, face-to-face: easiest if the woman has one foot up on a chair. Then she can turn around so now they are standing, his front to her back, again easier if she has one foot up on a chair. In another variation, she bends over to touch her toes (knees slightly bent to avoid strain) and he enters her from behind. Or she stands up and bends over the back of a sofa.

Then we get to doggie style, what I call "Fido and Fifi," after two poodles. She is in knee-chest position facing down, right at the edge of the bed, with her tush way up in the air. He is standing on the floor and he enters her from behind. This is also the best position if you are going to be involved in anal sex. It can also work if he is kneeling on the mattress, but his thrusting will be gentler.

Then there is good old *soixante-neuf,* or 69, head to genitals and genitals to head. This is not intercourse but great stimulation.

Let's not forget the old rocking chair or any sturdy chair. She sits on his lap facing him and puts his penis in her vagina, or she faces away from him, penis entering from behind.

There you go, fifteen tried-and-true sexual positions. Now some people in a new relationship, or people who are shy, modest, or embarrassed about their bodies, may not be comfortable trying these on for size.

There are a few great books with beautiful drawings that really do give permission to be innovative, and show how to just let go and have fun in bed: *Ultimate Sex* by Anne Hooper (New York: DK Publishing, 2001); *The Magic of Sex* by Miriam Stoppard (New York: Penguin, 2001); *Seduce Me: How to Ignite Your Partner's Passion* by Darcy A. Cole (Booklocker. com, 2003); or *The Complete Idiot's Guide to Amazing Sex* by Sari Locker (Indianapolis: Alpha Books, 2002), 2nd ed. Or go and get out that old copy of *The Joy of Sex* by Dr. Alex Comfort (New York: Crown, 2002), rev. ed.

POWER/CONTROL

Usually I do not have a handout for this topic, but this issue has come up repeatedly in the past months. It's tricky and can be complicated, because often a disagreement appears to be about one issue, but this issue is used to wield power and control over the other partner. It's time to take a look at this problem.

Dear Sue: *I have been married for five years, but even before that I had a male friend whom I really liked; we were dear, close friends, nothing more. My husband liked him, too, and included him in our activities. Last week my friend hesitantly told me he was gay, which did not upset me, I was okay. A few days later I told my husband. Big mistake—he lost it totally. Calling our friend all kinds of names, he told me I was not to see him or talk to him again.*

If my friend phones, my husband is very abrupt and says that I am out or that I am busy. I haven't told my friend. I don't know what to say.

Sue says: I agree, your good friend deserves an explanation, and to do anything less would be cruel. Would you consider writing him a very gentle letter explaining that your husband is having difficulty accepting this disclosure, and that you still love and want him as a friend but you will need a bit of time to help your husband work through his homophobia? Reassure your friend that you will contact him as soon as possible.

Then, without putting your husband on the defensive, try to find out why he is reacting this way. Could it be:

- He has homosexual fantasies.
- He is terrified your gay friend will make a pass at him and he will get involved?
- He thinks homosexuality is a perversion or a sin.
- He has a stereotypical image of a swishy, effeminate gay male and does not want to associate with a "pansy."

- Perhaps he was sexually abused by a male in his youth.

If you are able to gain some insight into his rejection of a friend, then you can be empathic, but you cannot act as his therapist. You don't have the counseling skills, nor can you stay detached, so he will need to see a therapist.

He may resist or refuse; if he does, simply tell him that you are having a great deal of difficulty dealing with this problem, it is beginning to affect your loving relationship, and you want to see a therapist. This is not to threaten him, but for yourself. I will be willing to bet that your husband will become involved before too long.

I must admit, I have some concerns here. Nobody has the right to dictate whom you may or may not be friends with. You are an adult, capable of deciding that for yourself. If your husband does not want to be involved, that is his decision, but he does not possess you.

I am concerned that this might escalate and that he might decide next that he does not like your mother. Then he could decide to move to a new community, far away from all your family and friends. This is the beginning pattern of abusers, and this could be classified as emotional abuse.

So you need to listen to his strong objections to your friendship and try to understand them. If you do not feel they are valid, if you are not willing to obey his command, then you must make that very clear to him. Tell him you are sorry he is upset, but that is clearly his problem and he is going to have to deal with it.

There is a great book that would be most helpful if he would read it. *Is It a Choice? Answers to 300 of the Most Commonly Asked Questions About Gays and Lesbians* by Eric Marcus (San Francisco: HarperSanFrancisco, 1999), rev. ed.

Dear Sue: *I have been going out with my boyfriend for over a year now. In the beginning I used to enjoy sex, although he wanted much more sex than I did. Now, after we have made love, he insists I go down on him. He pushes my head down and forces his penis into my mouth. If I refuse, he will say, "Please, please, just this once, it will only take a minute. I'm uncomfortable, I'll get lover's nuts if you don't relieve me."*

I used to like oral sex, but now I gag or I have an asthma attack. Afterward he is so sweet and so caring and always says, "Thank you, that was really nice." But I'm getting so I hate sex.

Sue says: Are we surprised? It is predictable that you would start avoiding sex altogether. If he insists, you will tense up, experience pain, and be turned right off. He will accuse you of being frigid or of having been with another guy; then he may find another female who is willing to satisfy him. Game over, score zero-zero. You may hate sex until you are able to figure out exactly the dynamics of this relationship. On the other hand, he may never figure out why you would break up, why all his relationships break up.

Can you learn how to communicate with him, not in the bedroom, but when you are out for a walk, or are doing the dishes? Tell him how you feel and how his behavior is affecting you. Then you must listen while he tells you what he needs (not pleading, begging, and beseeching). If you are sexually satisfied, then he needs to know that he can simply masturbate and satisfy himself.

Sounds so simple, but open, honest communication is a learned skill, and most of us did not learn it as we were growing up, so we really have to work at it.

Some books that stress communication are: *Creative Aggression: The Art of Assertive Living* by Dr. George R. Bach and Dr. Herb Goldberg (Gretna: Wellness Institute, 1974); *Don't Go Away Mad* by James Creighton, Ph.D. (New York: Doubleday, 1991). And you might benefit from *Couples: Exploring and Understanding the Cycles of Intimate Relationships* by Barry Dym, Ph.D., and Michael Glenn (New York: Perennial, 1994).

PREGNANCY

Pregnancy places more strain on a relationship than any other life experience. The crunch comes with the arrival of the new baby.

People frequently ask me questions about sex during and after pregnancy.

Dear Sue: *Is it safe to have sex while your partner is pregnant? Will it harm the baby?*

Sue says: Check it out with your doctor. If your partner does not have any bleeding or vaginal "show" (thick, bloody mucous discharge from her cervix), if she does not have any discomfort, and if she does not have a history of spontaneous or accidental abortions, she will be just fine.

The baby is well protected inside the dense muscular walls of the uterus, floating in a sac of amniotic fluid that acts as a shock absorber. A thick mucous plug in the cervix prevents infections from getting into the uterus, and your partner can't conceive yet another baby while she is pregnant, so again, she will be fine.

Some women feel glorious when pregnant, the epitome of femininity, and just love sex during pregnancy. Others feel fat and lumpy, out of shape, resentful that they have to go through this, and they do not want sex at all. Some of these feelings could be reduced if a woman gets lots of approval, acceptance, appreciation, and attention from her partner, and not only when he wants sex.

Many doctors used to recommend that during the last month of pregnancy you abstain from intercourse and that she not reach orgasm. Today, that is not the case for most couples. It takes a lot of creativity to have intercourse when she is eight and a half months pregnant, but imagination leads to great sex without intercourse.

Where there's a will, there's a way. Some couples use the female-on-top position, which works very well until the pregnancy is advanced. Probably the best position is the old favorite doggie style, with the woman resting on her arms and knees, tush up in the air, while he enters her vagina from behind. In this position, the heavy uterus falls forward and her abdomen is supported on the bed. He can manually stimulate her clitoris and it can be quite glorious.

You must admit, the image is humorous—all images of sex are pretty funny. If you can't laugh at sex, you shouldn't be doing it.

Two new warnings: pregnant women should not use a Jacuzzi or hot tub; the heat might trigger a miscarriage. Also, women who are planning on getting pregnant or who are already pregnant should not take ibuprofen for pain.

Dear Sue: I was so excited about my wife having a baby. I attended Lamaze classes, practiced coaching, and I was fine. But as we toured the delivery room, I broke into a cold sweat, started to feel sick, short of breath, and I thought I was going to faint. But real men don't do that, so I hung in there. When it came time to have the baby, she did well; I got through it, but I am a mess.

I felt so guilty about putting my wife through that much

pain! I could almost feel them doing the episiotomy, and I just about stained my britches when she was bearing down. I felt sick at the sight of the blood and the baby's head coming through. It was a nightmare that haunts me. As a result, I am reluctant to have sex with my wonderful wife. She thinks I don't find her attractive after the baby. It's not that, I just feel so guilty.

Sue says: Have you told your dearly beloved wife how you are feeling? She will probably not have the same memories at all. Sure it was hard work, sure it hurt, but she had your support, and now she has this beautiful baby; for her the delivery was all a blur. Personally, I'd rather have a baby than go to the dentist. Check it out with her; you may be putting yourself through this angst for no reason.

In any case, you're not alone. Pregnancy and childbirth can affect a couple's sex life. Some males really resent a male doctor touching their partner's genitals and delivering the baby, feeling that the doctor has a special relationship that he as a partner will never have. Now her genitals are no longer "his." In actual fact, her genitals never were his—they are hers alone.

Other males run into difficulty when their partner becomes "the mother of my child" and they put her up on a pedestal. She is untouchable, like the Virgin Mary, and no longer allowed to be a lusty lady.

The expectation that all men should be with their wives in the delivery room removes the freedom of choice. Some men (and some women) simply pass out at the sight of blood. Why do we make those people feel guilty and inadequate if they know that it will be an upsetting experience for them?

So, ladies, if your partner does not really want to be in the delivery room, it would be in your best interest to give him permission to sit this one out in the waiting room.

Dear Sue: *How soon after the baby is born can you have sex?*

Sue says: Depends if you have a private room . . . Macho joke, sorry. Seriously, most doctors will not give you a definite answer because there are so many variables.

- She must *want* to have sex. Many times she is simply exhausted with the increased demands on her energy from breast-feeding and being up all night with a colicky, crying baby. She may be feeling inadequate as a mother and perhaps resenting the lack of support and help from her partner.
- Her genitals must have healed and must be back to almost normal again before you have sex.
- Most women prefer to wait till the lochia (postpartum discharge) is finished, which takes about a month.
- Some people say it is a good idea to wait until she has had her six-week checkup.
- Six weeks are required post–cesarean section for complete healing before intercourse.
- Some time is required before the hormones present during pregnancy flip off and the hormones of lactation click in and balance. During this period of flux, there may not be much action.

Many women are less than pleased with their new body; some call it rounder and fuller, but most call it flabby and saggy. Breasts lose their bounce and may be tender, and the nipples become large and dark and leak milk. A woman's abdomen may become bulgy or pendulous. Combine that with stretch marks, varicose veins, and yes, maybe hemorrhoids. Is she feeling sexy? Hardly.

If you do resume sex, make sure you have a good method

of birth control; you probably do not want to have another baby in ten months.

She is going to need a lot of love, support, and reassurance that you love her changed body. She is also going to need a lot of help with the new baby, the housework, and the endless laundry. Do read on—this is a very common problem for many couples:

Dear Sue: *Ever since the baby was born my wife has had no sex drive at all. I'm lucky if we have sex once a month, compared to twice a week before. What happened?*

Sue says: First, she should have a checkup with her family doctor just to be sure everything is okay. She may not be convinced her method of birth control is adequate, so check that out. Does she have any pain, discomfort, or bleeding? If all is okay physically, before we go any further, consider the possibility of fatigue as a cause of low sex drive.

New babies need and demand a great deal of attention. Often, subsequent babies seem easier, possibly because the mother has given up on perfection and doing everything herself and is more willing to let her partner, mother, and neighbors help out.

So it is understandable that a first-time mom is absolutely exhausted. When she finally does fall into bed, along comes her partner with that amorous gleam in his eye, the copulatory gaze, as some would call it.

Another question: Is your partner depressed? Some new mothers suffer postpartum depression and have difficulty adjusting to the new baby.

If these are not the cause of low sex drive, then we need to look at the relationship. What is happening in the bedroom generally reflects what is happening outside the bedroom.

Many times when I am counseling couples who have this problem, they both say that the relationship is good and strong. But when we get into in-depth counseling, they both are astounded at all the anger and resentment that comes to the surface.

You will both find you can deal with these feelings much more effectively with the help of a marriage or sex counselor. In a relationship, partners may think they are honest, but they do know how to manipulate and control each other, so it is impossible to be your own relationship counselor. A skilled therapist will keep you on track and will make sure you listen to each other and that you integrate what you learn about each other into your relationship. A counselor can help you develop a plan of action to eliminate or deal with problems now. You will also learn how to solve problems in the future.

Getting into couples' counseling is scary because you feel vulnerable, powerless, and afraid that the dynamics of the relationship will change. The old way is not working, but it was at least familiar and predictable. This is the unknown and you may feel lost. But that is great because you can relearn a whole new way of being together, which can work wonders for each of you as an individual, as a couple, and as a family.

Yes, it is expensive, no question; but think, this is your life, your future relationship as a family, so it is probably the best investment you could possibly make. So get on it now.

While you try to find a counselor, read and discuss *When Partners Become Parents: The Big Life Change for Couples* by Carolyn Pape Cowan and Philip A. Cowan (Mahwah: Lawrence Erlbaum, 1999). Turn off the TV and take time to read this book aloud together and discuss it. Also, take a look at *Is There Sex After Kids?* by Ellen Kreidman (New York: St. Martin's, 1996).

PREMATURE EJACULATION

Dear Sue: *I have a great girlfriend, but when we have sex I always come too fast. What can I do?*

Sue says: Premature ejaculation is now called ejaculatory incompetence by sex therapists. I am noticing a dramatic increase in the number of letters from males concerned that they come too fast. Therapy designed to prevent this is based on the squeeze technique or the stop-start technique, which retrain the male to recognize his body's signal indicating ejaculatory inevitability.

Many factors contribute to premature ejaculation: stress, anxiety, unrealistic expectations, or early sexual experiences that were rushed because of fear of discovery or because the man was having sex with a prostitute who wanted to turn a fast trick. Many males learn to masturbate in a hurry to get it over with. This sets a pattern for rapid ejaculation that may be difficult to break later on.

Here is what you can try. Have your partner stimulate you, or stimulate yourself, until you have a full erection. Just before you ejaculate, you will be aware of a twinge that tells you that it's coming. Stop immediately, let the erection subside, and then restimulate to have another. The therapy seems to work for some males, but not for all, and I recommend you find a good therapist who can teach you the technique properly. Some doctors are prescribing Paxil and Zoloft as possible treatments for premature ejaculation. Others are recommending Paxil and Viagra together as a solution. Do talk to your doctor.

Until something better comes along, I suggest you masturbate beforehand to reduce the sexual tension. This way you will be slower and more laid-back with your partner. Another delaying tactic: try female on top so she can stop stimulation. And if you do ejaculate too soon, continue to stimulate your partner while you go through the refractory phase when nothing can trigger another erection. But after twenty minutes (it takes longer for mature males), a young male can have another erection and he is back in action again. By this time your partner is fully aroused and excited, and you are a winner.

Some men try to slow things down by using anesthetic creams, tranquilizers, or alcohol, elastic bands, or double condoms, none of which helps the anxiety, the overriding issue here.

You may need to get some help from a good sex therapist, but in the meantime, I recommend these books: *The Magic of Sex* by Miriam Stoppard (New York: Penguin, 2001); *The New Male Sexuality* by Bernie Zilbergeld, Ph.D. (New York: Bantam, 1999); and *For Each Other: Sharing Sexual Intimacy* by Lonnie Barbach, Ph.D. (New York: Signet, 2001), reissue.

PREMENSTRUAL SYNDROME

We can all relate to that cartoon of a snarling black cat saying, "I have PMS and a gun, any questions?" Even with that, premenstrual syndrome is receiving much less press than it did a few years ago. Now menopause has taken the limelight. Still, for those who suffer from PMS, the symptoms are very real. This letter tells us how miserable it can be.

Dear Sue: *For fifteen days of every month, I am a positive bitch. I have every symptom in the book, including rapid mood changes. I am exhausted, angry, not interested in anything, least of all sex. I feel bloated, headachy, and constipated. Not* *a pretty picture. You name it, I got it. Is there anything I can do before my husband leaves me for the duration?*

Sue says: Most doctors would diagnose PMS with any four of the above symptoms during your monthly cycle. Keep a daily calendar of your symptoms and moods for three months so that your doctor can establish if you have PMS or another problem.

You may not like this, but PMS seems to affect well-educated professional women who have high expectations and a high level of stress. PMS is more common among women whose marriage is under stress. Generally, the condition appears anytime when a woman is in her thirties and after she has had children. It is also very common in women who have been sexually abused as children.

There are more than two hundred signs and symptoms of PMS. Once you have listed all your symptoms—and don't worry if they make you sound like a hypochondriac—make an appointment with your doctor, who may refer you to a PMS clinic or instigate treatment. This is purely trial and error. If you are on the birth-control pill, the doctor may take you off; if you are not on it, he may suggest you take it. Recent research indicates that PMS responds well to low doses of Prozac. Ask your doctor about this.

There are some things you can do for yourself. Eliminate tea, coffee, chocolate, cola, and alcohol, and reduce your salt intake. Increase your daily intake of B-complex vitamins, including B_{12} and folic acid. Establish a regular exercise program every day, whether you want to or not. Treat yourself during the worst time—have a massage or a movie night. Be sure you get enough rest and try to reduce the stress level in your life. That means not planning an anniversary bash for your in-laws during your PMS cycle.

Your marriage may be showing signs of stress, and you

might both benefit from relationship counseling with a good therapist to reestablish intimate communications so you can problem-solve more effectively.

It may be small comfort, but PMS generally improves after ten years or menopause, whichever comes first. So, for the duration, you have to do everything you can to manage the condition yourself. There is a great book you might want to read: *PMS: Solving the Puzzle* by Linaya Hahn (Louisville: Chicago Spectrum Press, 1995).

Dear Sue: *Do men suffer from PMS? My boyfriend gets moody and has a short fuse at certain times of the month.*

Sue says: There is some research that indicates that males do have cycles that seem to be related to lunar cycles. This is inconclusive; there does not seem to be a consistent pattern, and there are certainly no suggestions as to cause or cure. So the best you can do is identify his pattern, talk about it, and modify your lifestyle as best you can. Your being supportive will make it easier for both of you to survive his "wrong time of the month."

PROLAPSED UTERUS

Dear Sue: *After fifty-eight years of active life, marriage, and four kids, I don't deserve this problem, but my uterus is literally falling out of my vagina.*

Sue says: It used to be called a "fallen womb" (as opposed to a "fallen woman"). I do hope you have had this checked by your family doctor, who should refer you to a gynecologist (a doctor who specializes in problems in the female reproductive system).

The muscles and ligaments that support the uterus in your pelvic girdle have literally let go, allowing your uterus to prolapse, or slide down, until your cervix is protruding from your vagina. Now, this is not life threatening, but it is a risk in that it makes you vulnerable to infection and irritation and, possibly, bleeding. And it does mean that you will have to push the cervix back up to the top of your vagina before sex would be comfortable. This kinda kills the romance.

The treatment is a surgery that involves taking other abdominal muscles and attaching them to the uterus to suspend it from the top of the vagina where it belongs. Or, the gynecologist may recommend a hysterectomy, or removal of the offending uterus (see page 144).

Some mature women are too embarrassed to discuss these types of problems with their doctor. However, most doctors are unflappable and are glad to provide advice and information. If you are still reluctant, do find yourself a nice friendly female doctor with whom you might be more comfortable discussing "private" matters concerning your health.

PROSTATE TUMORS

Dear Sue: *I must have surgery because they think I have a tumor on my prostate. Will it mean the end of my sex life forever?*

Sue says: Until recently, yes, it would have. A prostatectomy for cancer would always sever the nerves that triggered an erection. But now with transurethral resection of the prostate (TURP), a surgery for benign, non-cancerous tumors, the nerves, blood supply, and hormones are not affected. This means the surgery should not affect sexual function other than causing retrograde ejaculation. Thus the sensation of orgasm will remain the same, but because the prostatic valves will have been removed, the semen will be deposited in the bladder instead of being ejaculated.

About 25 percent of men who have had a TURP may experience some sexual problems as a result of anxiety and fear of erectile failure. Good pre- and post-operative counseling can be beneficial.

We have to acknowledge the connection between the brain and the "bod." If you are worried and convinced that you will never get it up again, no matter how good your surgeon is, that self-fulfilling prophecy will come true. You will have nocturnal and morning erections when your brain is shut off. If this is the case, you will realize you are making yourself impotent, at which point it would be time to find yourself a good sex therapist. Really, I kid you not. Now there are several new treatments that do not involve surgery. Do talk to a urologist to explore your options.

Dear Sue: My husband has been diagnosed with cancer of the prostate. I know it seems selfish, but I have heard that cancer may be caused by a virus. If so, I am scared that I could get cancer of the cervix or uterus from him because we have been having sex quite regularly. Should I be checked out?

Sue says: You are not at risk because your husband has cancer of the prostate. You can't catch cancer as you catch a cold or the flu. So please relax and enjoy.

However, for your own sake, do not ignore such changes in your body as bleeding, pain, lumps, swelling, shortness of breath, or bruising. Do continue to have your annual physical exam, including a breast and pelvic exam, not because you are at risk from your husband's condition, but just for your own health.

PROSTATIC STIMULATION

Dear Sue: *Is this gross or what? My husband finds it a real turn-on if I take a big gob of Vaseline and insert it into his anus, crook my fingers forward, and very gently rub something that feels like a small, soft nut in there. Is this normal? Will I hurt him? Does he have another undescended testicle?*

Sue says: No, no, and no to all your questions. This is called prostatic stimulation. You are very gently stroking the small gland that is wrapped around his urethra, the tube that carries urine from his bladder through his penis.

Some men just go ape over this type of stimulation—anatomically, the prostate gland is analogous to the G-spot of a female. They call it the A-spot. However, other men find it excruciatingly painful—it reminds them of the doctor doing a yearly physical exam.

The secret is clean hands and lots of lubrication. Vaseline is okay unless it comes in contact with a condom. Be very, very gentle, and don't do it too long or it will irritate him. You can buy latex gloves at the drugstore if you feel better that way, or slide a lubricated condom over your fingers.

No two males are alike—what is one man's pleasure is another man's torture. If you are comfortable with this behavior, it is harmless.

PROSTITUTION

Dear Sue: *Would you please give your listeners some insight into prostitution? We are not the sleazy ladies we are painted to be. We are sex workers in the sex trade.*

Sue says: Personally, I have no moral problem with prostitution, but I sure do have some concerns. There are many "pros," smart ladies and gents who are responsible, practice Safer Sex, take care of their health and safety, and perform a service that is not new on the market. They are professionals.

I have one letter from a gentleman who is married and he says he and his wife love each other and have sex regularly. But while most guys pick up a cup of coffee on their way to work every day, this man drives by one particular spot and picks up his regular "lady of the morning," she performs fellatio on him, he pays, and they part till tomorrow.

Now, we know oral sex is low-risk behavior, so he is probably safe. But I do have to wonder about his need for that kick start to his day—the rush he gets from doing something that could get him and this woman arrested, and that could affect the trust level of his relationship.

Of greater concern to me are teenage kids, often runaways, who survive by turning quick tricks for ten or fifteen dollars and do not always insist on a condom. They may also have turned to prostitution to support their drug habit. These kids, both males and females, are vulnerable to violence and being controlled by a pimp, who may get them hooked on drugs or beat them up if they don't turn enough tricks. This really does upset me.

There are some excellent community support groups for kids: Street Outreach Services, Covenant House, and many others. I do not have any answers here, but I do have concerns.

[r]

RELATIONSHIPS

There are so many excellent books available on relationships and communication that it would be pointless for me to try to cover all the convolutions and machinations of our intimate, loving connections. As a result, I am including some condensed insights and a book list so that you can choose what you want to read.

Dear Sue: *My girlfriend and I have a great relationship right now, but our friends are breaking up all around us. What can we do to keep our love alive?*

Sue says: This is a biggie. But you do know what you want, and you are willing to work on maintaining that sense of togetherness. You have already proved that you are capable of keeping the loving intimacy in your relationship. You can maintain a good relationship with your partner if you:

- Don't take your partner for granted.
- Check things out on a regular basis.
- Always consult your partner before you make a decision that involves her—invitations and family affairs.
- Be considerate, thoughtful, and sensitive to her needs.
- Practice good communication skills by using "I" terms. Saying "I feel hurt" instead of "you're hurting my feelings" will keep your partner from getting on the defensive. Continue with your empathic listening skills.
- Don't smother, control, or manipulate each other.
- Avoid becoming enmeshed in each other's life—allow your partner space and time to do her own thing. You need a balance of togetherness and separateness to maintain your own autonomy and individuality. Otherwise, the relationship controls you instead of you controlling the relationship.
- Give permission and encouragement to your partner to grow and develop while you do the same. This can be scary, because you do not know where it will lead and how you will fit into the new dynamic, which can be threatening. But everyone changes, so try on new behavior and incorporate what works well into your persona and reject what does not fit. The relationship is always evolving. This helps prevent monotony and boredom. Negotiate and solve problems as they come up.
- Conflicts that are not resolved will not go away. If they are swept under the carpet, they will build up and eventually give rise to a nasty argument. What you resist, persists.
- Do continue to be romantic and woo your partner. Express warm, tender, loving feelings that let her

know you think she is special. Again, the essential components of a loving relationship are the four big As: attention, approval, appreciation, and acceptance.
- Be prepared for the ups and downs that will happen in any relationship. Tell your partner when you are concerned or scared and discuss the best way to get through your downers.
- If you find that things are coming apart at the seams, do not just hope that the problems will go away. Get relationship counseling and read some books together.
- Trust your partner, trust your relationship, and share the determination to make it last.

Even if you and your partner are able to implement these suggestions into your daily life, there will be arguments and disagreements:

Dear Sue: *I have been married for twenty-five years and it has been fine. But now I feel angry with my husband a lot of the time, and I am critical and faultfinding. He just doesn't get it. How can I convince him that I want things to change?*

Sue says: We all develop defense mechanisms to avoid having to deal with conflicts. There are many avoidance techniques.

- Giving in without a fight or changing behavior patterns for a short time and then gradually sliding back into the old ways.
- Agreeing that there is a problem, but postponing any action to deal with it.
- Bluster, bravado, and overreacting to intimidate and scare your partner into dropping an issue. Saying

things like, "Right, that's it. Let's just call it quits and get a divorce."

- Sticking your head in the sand and hoping it will all blow over.
- Playing dumb and pretending not to understand what your partner is talking about.
- Criticizing and putting your partner down: "That's stupid."
- Shifting blame onto your partner or onto somebody else, anybody but yourself.
- Taking the martyr attitude: "You're right, I'm a dud and you deserve better."

People develop these avoidance techniques and then mix and match them, anything to keep their partners off balance so they can deny, delay, or avoid making changes that might disrupt the balance of power.

In a book called *The Games People Play,* published in the early seventies, Eric Berne outlined most of the strategies people unconsciously use to deal with conflict. When you learn the name of the game, you find the antithesis or antidote to counteract the game and use it. It's devious, but it works.

A more honest approach would be to name the game, but not to lay blame on the player. No matter which avoidance tactic your partner employs, you can stop and simply use "I" terms ("I have difficulty discussing this," or "I am reluctant to get into a discussion because I feel I am being manipulated").

There is no point in saying, "You always do X," because the other person will say, "No, I don't—" and that's that, and you come out as the nagging Witch of the West. On the other hand, if you put it in terms of "I feel—," your partner can say, "Don't be silly," but cannot deny you your feelings. They are yours and they are valid.

Here are a number of books I recommend: *Intimacy* by Dan McAdams (New York: Doubleday, 1989); *Loving Him Without Losing You* by Carolyn Nordon Bushong (New York: Berkley, 1993); *Will He Love Me Forever? Sustaining Love through the Years* by Julian D. Ford and Judith G. Ford (New York: McGraw-Hill, 1991); *Rekindling Desire: Bringing Your Sexual Relationship to Life* by Warwick Williams (Oakland, Calif.: New Harbinger Publications, 1988); *Couples: Exploring and Understanding the Cycles of Intimate Relationships* by Barry Dym, Ph.D., and Michael Glenn (New York: Perennial, 1994); *My Enemy, My Love: Man-Hating and Ambivalence in Women's Lives* by Judith Levine (New York: Anchor, 1993); *When I Say No, I Feel Guilty* by Manuel J. Smith (New York: Bantam Books, 1985); *Boys Will Be Boys* by Myriam Miedzian (New York: Doubleday, 1991); *Going the Distance: Finding and Keeping Lifelong Love* by Lonnie Barbach and David L. Geisinger (New York: Plume, 1993); *Intimate Connections* by David D. Burns, M.D. (New York: NAL, 1986); *The Intimate Enemy: How to Fight Fair in Love and Marriage* by George R. Bach and Peter Wyden (New York: Avon, 1983); *Genderspeak: Men, Women and the Gentle Art of Verbal Self-Defense* by Suzette Hayden Elgin (New York: Wiley, 1993).

RETARDED (DELAYED) EJACULATION

About 4 percent of males may experience retarded, or delayed, ejaculation.

Dear Sue: *My husband simply cannot ejaculate near me. So far, that has been okay because he has strong erections and can last forever, and when I am satisfied, he simply mastur-*

bates and he is fine. No problem—except, now we want to have a baby, and it just ain't gonna happen this way.

Sue says: This should be no problem for you because you are both comfortable with your bodies and your sexuality, but for some people these suggestions would be unacceptable.

I suggest that you and your partner really take a look at the possible reasons he is unable to ejaculate with you around. If he is able to masturbate and ejaculate all by himself, then there is nothing physically wrong, but a psychological barrier is stopping him. These barriers are usually based on fear: fear of getting a disease, hurting you, getting you pregnant, getting caught by parents, becoming trapped in your vagina. Perhaps he finds genital odors a real turnoff. You would probably both benefit from visiting a good sex therapist. My fear is that in time, you may feel rejected, or feel that there is something wrong with you or that he does not love you anymore, or that he thinks sex is dirty.

Meanwhile, if you want to get pregnant, you have to figure out a way to get his ejaculate into your vagina. First, get out the calendar and work out exactly when you should be ovulating. At that time, have sex the way you usually do, but have your partner wear a condom when he masturbates and ejaculates. Then you lie on your back, take the condom, place the open end into your vagina, and squeeze out all the ejaculate.

If that is too squishy for you, he can ejaculate into a clean jam jar; then you can get out the old turkey baster, and squeeze the bulb to get suction. Insert the nozzle into the ejaculate, release the collapsed bulb to draw the ejaculate up into the tube. Then gently insert the tube into your vagina as close to your cervix as possible, squeeze the bulb, and deposit the ejaculate, which contains millions of sperm, into your vagina. Elevate your hips on a couple of pillows and stay there for about an hour to give the sperm the best exposure possible. Lotsa luck.

I suggest you and your husband read these books together: *The New Male Sexuality* by Bernie Zilbergeld, Ph.D. (New York: Bantam, 1999), and *The Magic of Sex* by Miriam Stoppard (New York: Penguin, 2001).

[s]

SELF-CONCEPT, SELF-ESTEEM

There are two components to self-image: self-concept and self-esteem. Self-concept is about the questions "Who am I? How do I see myself?" Self-esteem is about "What am I worth and how do other people see me? Where do I fit in to the scheme of things?"

It is pretty hard to develop a good self-concept and self-esteem if you have been raised in a toxic family such as this one:

Dear Sue: I don't know where to turn for help. I am so alone—no family, no friends. All my life I have been put down and teased. I'm quiet, a "browner," not because I am that smart, but I spent all my time in my bedroom studying to get away from my mother, her assorted lovers, and an older cousin who lived with us and took great delight in punching me out. I just can't seem to get anything right, so I simply with-draw, but I wish I was like all the other kids.

Sue says: Although I would not want you to be "like all the other kids," I would love to be able to give you a shot of chutzpah so the real you could emerge and join the other kids.

Unfortunately there is no quick fix here. You have experienced a great deal of emotional, and even physical, abuse. You won't get over it the day after tomorrow.

Please realize that this is not something you can get over alone. You will need some counseling. Check out the guidance counseling service at your school. Perhaps your family doctor can suggest a counselor or can refer you to a mental health clinic at your local hospital. You can also ask your school nurse, minister, or family services organization about getting help.

While you are waiting for an appointment, there are a few things you can do for yourself. Purchase an inexpensive notebook, which will become your own personal journal. Brainstorm and jot down all your strong points. Don't be bashful—you are not boasting, but you are acknowledging the talents and assets you have. They may be a sense of humor or great legs. You will come to accept these assets and use them to reinforce other wobbly areas or build up new areas of competence, self-concept, and self-esteem. This is empowering.

You will notice that negatives and put-downs are not as devastating as they once were when you develop the ability to put them into perspective or reject them outright. You will develop coping skills and soon you will take that one step further. When someone tries to belittle you, you will decide, "I don't need that kind of treatment. I deserve better than that, and I am not going to allow you to negate me."

You can develop one-liners like "I really needed to hear that," or "I can always count on you to try to make me feel bad." Think about Eleanor Roosevelt's statement, "No one can make you feel bad without your permission."

There is one activity we all engage in, but we deny we do it, even if it helps us: self-talk. Stuck in a traffic jam, we mutter to ourselves to reinforce the positive or negative affirmations we have received. Make your self-talk positive.

There is another journal strategy you might want to try. Develop a five-year plan for your life—where you want to be at that point, what you want out of life. No matter how far out it seems, jot it down. Then make a wish list in order of priorities to develop a plan that will move you toward your goal. By doing this, you will be moving from wishful thinking to making what you want a reality.

Now you may notice that you are starting to take some risks. You are less fearful and are developing a sense of yourself as a person, feeling competent and capable and willing to take risks, such as making friends, trying different hobbies, sports, and other pastimes.

True self-concept and self-esteem will not permit you to manipulate, coerce, intimidate, or threaten anybody else. That kind of behavior stems from a low self-image.

Studies have shown that parents who have high self-esteem communicate that to their children. Their kids become independent and self-sufficient, make good decisions for themselves, and require less discipline. They also have good relationships with their family and friends.

Initially, self-concept comes from parents, then from the extended family, day care, and school. Females' self-image takes a nosedive during adolescence when they may have acne, small breasts, irregular, heavy periods, greasy hair, and baby fat. They watch *The O.C.*, read *Seventeen* magazine, and look at Britney Spears and Christina Aguilera as embodying an ideal they will never attain.

A male may feel like a runt and a total klutz, with no social skills and a body that produces continual spontaneous erections, which make him feel like an oversexed pervert.

Our goal is to raise kids to be competent, cooperative, and decisive. Parents and teachers can help raise self-concept in a number of ways.

- Give praise and encouragement to all kids. Emphasize what they can do. Give them permission to try things. If they fail, tell them it's okay, they'll do better next time. The six critical messages that all kids need to hear regularly when they are growing up are: "I believe in you"; "I trust you"; "I know you can handle it"; "I hear you"; "I care about you"; "You are important."
- Do not tease kids, put them down, or make fun of their goofs.
- Make information easily available. Teach kids how to access information and answer all questions honestly.
- Offer kindness, consideration, and open communication.
- Help kids become assertive, not obnoxiously aggressive. Encourage them to bring up feelings and concerns, knowing they will be dealt with fairly. This way they do not become doormats for the world.

SEX ADDICTION

Sex addiction is a controversial and complicated obsessive-compulsive behavior, as this letter indicates.

Dear Sue: *I am a twenty-six-year-old male with a high sex drive and emotion-control problem. For the past two years I have been dating an extremely gorgeous, sexy blonde, and we both really got off on sex. Then my sex drive got out of whack; it consumed my life and took priority over everything else. She started to chill out and was less enthusiastic since I was after her every moment. After sex, she could just go to sleep. I was an animal. I wanted more.*

So I would get up, go to a bar, pick up some woman, and have more sex. One night my girlfriend followed me, and that was it. She said, "Get help or get out." Where do I go?

Sue says: Some therapists say that sexual addiction is simply an excuse to justify lack of control and unwillingness to conform to acceptable norms.

Other psychiatrists and psychologists maintain that it is a compulsive behavior that has its roots in early childhood and can afflict both males and females. It is believed that people who suffer from this disorder come from dysfunctional families that failed to provide security or to reinforce the child's self-concept and self-esteem, and in which there was an absence of trust. The child felt empty, abandoned, and vulnerable. There is evidence that a high percentage of people who experience the need to have continuous compulsive sex were physically or emotionally abused as children.

Generally, these children were brought up to believe sex was shameful, and that fantasizing and masturbation were unacceptable. They also did not develop social or dating skills.

An intricate psychological pattern seems to emerge when they become adults. These people are involved in sex, which provides temporary relief that turns into disgust with themselves, shame, and anxiety. They then become determined to avoid sexual contact, which results in overcontrol that cannot be sustained. They experience an inability to cope, the upshot of which is that they seek a sexual "fix" again, bringing them back to square one.

Once we see the pattern, we can identify some of the characteristics of sexually compulsive behavior.

- Desire for attention.
- Risk taking, looking for a high, a fix, an escape from boredom or emptiness, pleasure with no emotional involvement.
- Anger and rage at women or at themselves for being inadequate.
- Desire to be punished—"I'm a bad person"—and low self-image.
- Desire for power and control when they are feeling powerless and out of control in their personal lives.

So you can see that this is not just a case of being "out-of-control horny." This is a serious psychological problem, and I think that you would benefit from in-depth counseling. Psychiatrists are finding that high doses of Prozac are beneficial in conjunction with psychotherapy.

There will be some relationship issues that you will have to resolve—this is simply not something that you can forgive and forget. You will have to gain insight into the cause of your behavior and the effect it has had on your relationship; then do some personal healing. We are talking individual and conjoint relationship counseling focusing on forgiveness to reestablish trust. You may both need help in dealing with sexual problems that can arise out of this addiction. In many major cities in North America there is an organization called Sex and Love Addicts Anonymous (SLAA).

There are some excellent books for you to read: *Don't Call It Love* by Patrick Carnes (New York: Bantam, 1992); *Love and Addiction* by Stanton Peel and Archie Brodsky (New York: Signet, 1981); and *Escape from Intimacy: Untangling the "Love" Addictions—Sex, Romance, Relationships* by Anne Wilson Schaef (San Francisco: Harper San Francisco, 1990).

SEXUAL ASSAULT

We used to call it rape. Nowadays, it is classed as sexual assault, but women who are victims still call it rape. When we say the word "rape," the visual image that flashes into our mind is of being grabbed from behind by an unknown assailant, dragged into an underground parking garage, and forced to submit to intercourse against our will. And yes, that does still happen.

A woman shares her experiences in this letter:

Dear Sue: *I was home alone, in bed, sound asleep, when I woke up feeling a person holding a knife to my throat, who threatened to kill me if I moved. Using the knife, he cut off my nightie, tried to put his penis in my vagina, but he went limp, so he forced me to perform oral sex on him till he had an erection. Then he rolled me over and forced his penis into my bum. After he left, I cried and cried in the tub. Then I went to the emergency room. They were so fantastic. A woman from the rape crisis center stayed with me. I moved and settled into a new apartment. Then I went for individual counseling and group therapy. Now, five years later, I am okay, but occasionally I have nightmares, and I am nervous if I am alone at night.*

Fortunately, I have a wonderful boyfriend who is very understanding and patient with me. Usually I am okay with sex, but every once in a while, if he moves a certain way, a cer tain sound or smell can trigger memories and I freeze. I am still in therapy and it is getting better, but I sometimes wonder if I will ever be able to put it all behind me.

Sue says: We can just feel the terror as you describe this horrific sexual assault. It is terrifying and degrading, and we feel violated and afraid to go out. The thought of sex may be repulsive. It is fortunate that you have counseling, and that your partner is supportive and caring. You have a good chance of being a winner.

There are so many horror stories of abuse, mostly about women, but males may also be sexually assaulted, occasionally by parents or by older siblings or other members of their extended family. Most often, young men or boys are assaulted by older males who are friends or well known to the victim.

Dear Sue: *I was a member of a club. We were camping and there was no room in the other guys' tent, so I had to sleep in the leader's tent. In the middle of the night, he climbed into my sleeping bag, fondled my penis, and forced me to perform oral sex on him. He also sucked on mine. When we got home, I told my mom, who reported him to the police. The publicity was awful. He was charged but found not guilty; he resigned from the group, and I looked like a fool. Since then I have not been able to trust any man, and I have trouble with sexual relationships. I also have insomnia and nightmares. Friends think I must be gay, but I know I am not homosexual. Help—*

Sue says: Males are reluctant to report sexual assault because they feel no one will believe them, or that they may be regarded as a wimp: "Why didn't you fight or run away?" People might say, "If you were a real man, you would have enjoyed it," or "It happened, now get over it."

So guys are reluctant to disclose abuse unless they are in severe distress. They experience many of the same signs and symptoms as women do, plus a few that are unique to males. They feel different; they become loners, outsiders; they do not trust others and have difficulty being involved in an intimate relationship. Sex may be a chore. They are not able to be spontaneous, playful, or have fun; or they may question their sexual orientation, have poor social skills, and expect to be hurt so that it becomes a self-fulfilling prophecy, or they may deny all feelings, including love and intimacy. Again, drug and alcohol abuse may become a problem.

I have had a great deal of difficulty finding good counseling and therapists for males who were sexually abused as children. There are few support groups and few books specifically for males. However, these two books may help you: *Victims No Longer: Men Recovering from Incest and Other Sexual Child Abuse* by Mike Lew (New York: Perennial, 1990); *Broken Boys—Mending Men: Recovery from Childhood Sexual Abuse* by Stephen D. Grubman-Black (Caldwell: The Blackburn Press, 2002).

Dear Sue: *My husband has been posted overseas for six months and is due home in a few weeks. About a month ago after work one day, another employee and I went out for a drink together, which turned into dinner. Then we went back to his place to look at his wedding pictures. All of a sudden, he started to undress me and forced me to have sex, using no protection whatsoever. I was so embarrassed and ashamed that I did not tell anybody, but I feel dirty and angry with him and with me. I definitely will not tell my husband when he comes home. He would hold it against me forever. I am scared that I won't want him to touch me because the thought of sex makes me physically ill. Fortu-*

nately, I'm on the Pill, but what if I got HIV/AIDS from this jerk?

Sue says: You will probably feel better once you develop a plan of action and start implementing it. Go to your family doctor and explain what happened. Have the tests for STIs. While you are there, ask for a referral to a therapist or counselor to help you work through some of your feelings of anger, guilt, shame, and your revulsion against sex. Go to the library or bookstore and gather all the helpful books about sexual assault that you can find. I think it would be beneficial if you could start keeping a journal of your feelings.

Clearly, you have decided not to tell your husband about the assault, but you may wish to rethink that decision. In your journal, write out a dialogue that you could use to disclose what happened. Also, list exactly how you think he might react if he knew, and reassess whether it would not be easier in the long run to tell him just what happened. Then you could both get relationship counseling to work through all the feelings. Keeping this a big secret can certainly get complicated, and if he ever did find out, the trust level in your relationship would be seriously damaged.

Now, if you simply cannot (meaning "will not") tell him, and you still have this overriding concern about HIV/AIDS, you will not be able to get an accurate test for HIV until fourteen weeks after the assault took place. Hubby is due home in two weeks, so you have to find some way to get him to agree to Safer Sex without arousing his suspicions. I can think of only one excuse you could use: you could say the doctor took you off the birth-control pill for a few months because you were having problems on the Pill, and you do not want to get pregnant right now, so the best bet is to use condoms. When the "window period" (see page 19 on HIV/AIDS) has passed, you can be tested, wait two weeks for the results, and when they come back negative, you can give the all-clear signal and stop using condoms.

I still prefer honesty in a relationship, but you know your husband and you have to do what you think would be best. Lotsa luck. Do continue with counseling until you are able to enjoy the sexual component of your marriage.

It is not possible to cover the topic of sexual assault in depth in this book, but many good books are available that are helpful. I encourage you to keep a journal and get individual counseling and find a support group to help you move beyond the personal pain.

SEXUALLY TRANSMITTED DISEASES

Chlamydia

Dear Sue: *I have a new boyfriend, and we had sex without a condom. I decided to go on the Pill, and the doctor did routine tests. They called me a few days later and told me I had chlamydia. What is it?*

Sue says: Chlamydia is a serious sexually transmitted disease that is two or three times more common than gonorrhea. It is spread by sexual contact, including oral-genital sex. Symptoms, which may develop in seven to twenty-one days, include a clear discharge and pain during urination or during sex. However, generally 70 percent of women and 10 percent of males have no signs or symptoms. For every male who has chlamydia, there are ten women who are infected.

If the infection is not treated in women, infection in the fallopian tubes can develop, which, if not treated, will result in sterility. If these infections spread, pelvic inflammatory dis ease (PID) results, requiring hospitalization. PID may result in an increased risk of ectopic pregnancy or sterility. If a woman has chlamydia when she delivers a baby, the baby might develop eye infections or pneumonia. This is why the law requires that all babies be given antibiotic drops in their eyes at birth. Untreated in males, chlamydia may result in sterility.

Testing for chlamydia is not done routinely, unless there are symptoms, or unless you specifically request to be tested. A swab is taken from the cervix in women or the urethra (the opening of the penis) in males. If one of the partners has chlamydia, the other would automatically be treated. Testing is not painful (and, if you're Canadian, is automatically covered by your provincial health plan). Go to an STD clinic or your family doctor.

Treatment consists of oral antibiotics for ten days. Do take all the medication as prescribed and abstain from sex until you're retested and cured.

The best protections, the only protections, are to abstain from sex, have a strictly monogamous relationship, or use a condom. Even with this, women should ask to be tested for chlamydia during their annual medical checkup.

Gonorrhea

Dear Sue: *This is really embarrassing, but I met a woman in a bar, and we went back to my place, where we had sex, no condom. Not smart. About four days later, I had a very small amount of discharge and a bit of burning, especially when I peed. I went to an STI clinic and found out I had "clap." They gave me the treatment right away and it is all gone now, but they want me back. Why? They were very determined to get the lady's name, so I went back to the bar and met her again,* *got her name, and told her I got a disease from her. She denied it. Now what?*

Sue says: *Clap* is slang for "gonorrhea." You contracted it from unprotected sex with this lady. You were lucky because you got the symptoms—the discharge, which is actually pus, and the burning when you started and stopped urinating. Some males also notice that they have "frequency" (an urge to urinate more frequently than normal). Many times there are no signs and symptoms, as in the case of your lady friend. People can have gonorrhea without even knowing they have it and spread it around quite easily.

Fortunately, you chose to go to a clinic to have this diagnosed. The staff does the testing and provides the gonorrhea medication free of charge, and they will want to retest you in three weeks to be sure you are cured. There are penicillin-resistant strains of gonorrhea around, so this is important. Do go. And do not have sex until you are retested and they tell you it's all clear. Tests for syphilis should also be done two to six months later (not to mention HIV).

Yes, doctors and STI clinics will insist that you locate your contact person(s). Otherwise, they could continue on their merry way and infect numerous other people. Once you disclosed the woman's name, they would very discreetly inform her that she should be tested and get treatment, and then they would try to locate the person who gave her the infection and any others whom she might have infected.

Women are more vulnerable to gonorrhea than man and may have no symptoms, so even though she denied she infected you, she should appreciate your contacting her. One hopes she will go to a doctor or clinic on her own, but your clinic would do a follow-up because untreated gonorrhea can develop into pelvic inflammatory disease (PID), which can cause sterility or, possibly, death. If she is pregnant and has gonorrhea when she goes into labor, the bacteria in her vagina could get into the baby's eyes during delivery. If the disease is not treated, it could cause blindness. Again, this is the reason babies have drops put in their eyes immediately after birth.

Had you been allergic to penicillin, another oral antibiotic would have been prescribed. Now, please do not think you can treat yourself with whatever you have in your medicine cabinet. Treatment for clap is two oral antibiotics taken immediately, and a follow-up. Go to a doctor or clinic.

Where you pulled your big boo-boo was not using a condom to protect yourself when you had sex with a stranger. I am willing to bet you will never do that again. Always carry condoms (but not in your wallet) and practice Safer Sex.

Hepatitis B

Dear Sue: *My boyfriend is just coming back from a round-the-world tour and he has hepatitis B. Should I worry?*

Sue says: Not to worry, but do ask your doctor where you can get a free injection, or find out if your extra-coverage health insurance from your job will pay for you to get a free immunization vaccination. That will protect you.

The hepatitis-B virus is not spread by food or water or casual kissing, but it is spread by sexual contact and intravenous drug users sharing needles. Medical and dental personnel who treat infected patients can also get it. Newborns whose mothers carry the virus may be infected and must be treated immediately after birth. Hepatitis B virus, or HBV, is rarely serious, but your boyfriend will need to take it easy for about four to six weeks. He will probably be chronically tired, jaundiced, and nauseated. He will also vomit and have no appetite, and will lose some weight as a result. Then he will be fine, although there is a small possibility that the virus might remain in his system and could infect you. A small number of patients get chronic active hepatitis, which may cause serious problems. So get the immunization to protect yourself.

In some diseases, such as HIV/AIDS and hepatitis B, the virus is very concentrated in a person's blood. So if you share needles and syringes, you are at high risk unless you rinse the needle and syringe with a weak solution of bleach in water, and then rinse it all in clear water before using it. Any way you look at it, doing heavy-duty drugs is risky business.

For more information on hepatitis B, contact the Hepatitis B Foundation, 700 E. Butler Ave., Doylestown, PA 18901; phone 215-489-4900; fax 215-489-4920; www.hepb.org.

Herpes Simplex

One of the worst things you could hear just after you have had sex: "That? Oh, that's just a blister." Panic time.

Dear Sue: *I have this very painful oozing blister on my penis. I had unprotected anal sex about a week ago. She said she was on the Pill, so I did not worry about birth control, and didn't use a condom. I thought bum sex was okay.*

Sue says: We cannot make a diagnosis sight unseen and without tests, but it could be herpes. Make an appointment with your doctor immediately for an examination while you still have this blister. If you prefer, you can find a sexually transmitted infection (STI) clinic through your department of

[253]

public health. Testing is free, but you will have to pay for medication.

There are different forms of the herpes virus, but simplex 1 and 2 are responsible for genital infection from sexual contact only. You do not get this from toilet seats, drinking fountains, or doorknobs. If you have nude genital sexual contact with a partner who has active lesions, the virus can be transmitted to you. It takes three to seven days before you notice the prodromal (early warning) symptoms. The first bout of herpes is always the worst; you may feel just awful—tired, headachy, nauseated, and you may notice an unusual blister on your genital area. It itches and burns so that you want to scratch, but it hurts.

Depending on the location of the lesion, you may experience pain and difficulty urinating. Sitting is uncomfortable and the friction of walking is agony. Really, you just want to lie down with a cool fan blowing on your genitals. The worst is over after four days, but it takes ten days to heal. There will not be a scar, but if you do have another outbreak, it will be in the same location.

The doctor can prescribe acyclovir cream, which may be effective for some, but not for most. From the onset of the prodromal symptoms and all the while you have this lesion, you must abstain from all sexual contact because you can infect your partner.

Herpes is caused by a virus that cannot be cured, and it stays in your system until you are under stress or a dramatic change in your life occurs, when you may experience symptoms. Suntanning and certain foods may trigger an outbreak. Some people have one outbreak and never have another. Some women have an outbreak with the onset of every menstrual period. The first attack is the worst. After that the outbreaks seem to be less severe, shorter, and less frequent.

There is oral medication available that is expensive but works very well for some people. It may be taken either one of two ways. Low-dose acyclovir pills may be taken every day to prevent an outbreak, or you can wait till you become aware of the prodromal symptoms and take larger doses for ten days. This will dramatically reduce the severity and the length of the outbreak.

If a woman is pregnant and has a history of frequent severe outbreaks of genital herpes, she must inform her doctor, who may recommend a cesarian section to prevent the baby's exposure to the virus.

Please note: if your partner has a cold sore on the mouth and you kiss her or him, you can develop cold sores, too. The herpes virus is spread by skin-to-skin contact. Also, if you perform oral-genital sex with your partner and you have a cold sore on your lip, you can transmit that virus and infect their genitals. And if your partner has an active genital-herpes lesion and you have oral sex, you can get it on your lip. Not a pretty sight.

Do read *The Truth About Herpes* by Dr. Stephen Sacks (Vancouver: Gordon Soules, 1997), 4th ed. You may have to order this book through your local bookstore, but it is the best book available and worth the wait.

There are herpes support groups in every major city, so do contact your department of health or Planned Parenthood to locate one near you.

Prevention is important. Have open, honest communication about all STIs before you engage in sex, and you must practice Safer Sex, using a condom every time. The new female condom will help protect female genitals because it covers most of a woman's external genitals. This will also protect male genitals if she has a herpes lesion around her genitals.

Venereal Warts

Dear Sue: *Tell me, can you get genital warts if your partner has a wart on his finger?*

Sue says: Genital warts are also called venereal warts. They are caused by a specific strain of the human papilloma virus. This is different from the virus that causes finger warts and plantar warts on your feet.

Genital warts are sexually transmitted and, again, you do not get them from toilet seats. The virus spreads by skin-to-skin contact, so if you have intimate sex with an infected partner, you are at risk. Problem: if you have had more than one partner, you may not know which one infected you; the virus may lie dormant, and you cannot know exactly how long you've had it.

It would be difficult for you to diagnose whether you have venereal warts, so see a doctor. Once you have had them, you know when they flare up. These warts are small, slightly raised, painless, pink-gray bumps that may appear on a woman's labia, around her rectum, or up in the vagina, where she would not see them. They may appear on the shaft or head of a man's penis, or they may be hiding under his foreskin, testicles, or around his rectum. Because a male's genitals are external, he is more liable to see these strange new bumps and go for a checkup. If they are diagnosed, he must tell his partner. Venereal warts may be precancerous if they are located in a woman's vagina or on her cervix.

There are several very effective treatments. If the warts are not too extensive, your doctor may "paint" them with a drug called podophyllin. This is allowed to dry and is left on for four hours. Then you must wash the solution off with soap and water, and you are fine. Allow it to heal for a few days. No sex. Sorry, but you are vulnerable; so is your partner.

Go back to the doctor, who may treat you again unless the warts have disappeared. Then you must use condoms for some time, and your partner must be treated and pronounced cured.

Some doctors spray liquid nitrogen on the warts; some use laser treatment, particularly if the warts are in the vagina. And some doctors surgically remove the warts if they have really spread.

The only way to guarantee protection is by not having sex. If you do have sex, make sure you and your partner have open, honest communication so you would be informed if there was an infection. And, do practice Safer Sex—use condoms.

For questions about *any* sexually transmitted disease, do check out *The Gynecological Sourcebook* by M. Sara Rosenthal (New York: McGraw-Hill, 2003), 4th ed.

SEX TOYS

Ben Wah Balls

Dear Sue: *What are ben wah balls? Do guys use them?*

Sue says: Balls are not new. They originated in Asian countries and have recently been imported into North America. They are one-inch-round stainless-steel balls that females may insert into their vagina during the day, and as they move, they create sexual stimulation. To retain the balls, women develop very strong pubococcygeal muscles just as they would when practicing Kegel exercises. This increases the sexual pleasure of both partners. The balls are easy to remove and can be washed.

Occasionally males inquire about using ben wah balls in their rectum. Retrieving them may be a problem, so some guys put the balls in the toe of a nylon knee-high panty hose. Using lots and lots of lubrication, they gently insert the balls into their rectum with the top of the stocking extending outside the body. The operative words here are "lots of lubrication." And I would not recommend this if you have hemorrhoids. Inserting and removing the balls could aggravate the piles.

Do be sure to wash all sex toys well between each partner and after each time you use them.

Vibrators

Dear Sue: *My boyfriend was posted overseas, so as a joke, he bought me a vibrator as a going-away gift. I must confess, I became very proficient at using it. Now that he is home, he has become very attached to my vibrator. He likes me to use it while we are having sex, not only on me but on him. He loves it if I use it to touch his testicles and around his rectum. Does he like my vibrator better than me?*

Sue says: What a wonderful question. You seem to be feeling inadequate, threatened by a battery-operated gizmo instead of seeing it as a toy. You question your attractiveness and ability as a lover. In reality, you can see the whole thing as a compliment. In a playful way, he cared enough about you to give you this thoughtful gift, and now he is secure enough in your relationship and in his sexual skills that he is comfortable using the vibrator along with his penis to pleasure both of you. Think about this. Did you become so addicted to the vibrator that you were not interested in him? No. Then what makes you think you will be displaced by a vibrator?

Just be sure to keep the batteries charged! And a further word about vibrators. They are fine and fun, but they must be washed after every use to reduce the risk of transmitting infection. Also, if you use them for anal stimulation, you must either use a condom over them or wash them well before using them for vaginal stimulation.

There are wonderful vibrators available that have been designed to look like the real thing. This can add a whole new twist to making love. A dildo also looks like a penis, but is usually hard, rigid, and does not vibrate.

Contrary to what males believe, most females do not use a vibrator to mimic the thrusting actions of a penis during intercourse. Most women use a vibrator to provide breast and genital stimulation, focusing on the clitoris, around the vagina opening, and perhaps thrusting.

Before you run out and invest thirty-five dollars in this sex toy, check it out with your partner. You could say, "The guys [girls] at work were joking about using a vibrator and one guy said he and his wife loved using it. It sounded like fun. How would you feel about trying it the next time we get together?"

They are available from most specialty shops, or by catalog, if you are shy. Also, take a look at this wonderful book: *The Many Joys of Sex Toys* by Anne Seman (New York Broadway, 2004), which is coming out in fall 2004.

SHY MAN SYNDROME

Dear Sue: *I am a thirty-five-year-old male, presentable, shy, well educated, with an MBA. I meet a lot of very attractive women at work, but I just can't approach them for a date. I desperately want to get married, have a family, and live a normal life.*

Sue says: You seem like every woman's dream come true, except that it may not happen. Perhaps you are experiencing what we call "shy man syndrome." If we checked further we would probably find that your mother is an outspoken, strong character who is critical of everybody and into put-downs in a subtle way.

There are other characteristics of men who are love-shy:

- Their father is quiet, withdrawn, and not too involved in parenting.
- They probably have several gregarious brothers and no sisters, so they end up with a distorted picture of females, with no idea how to approach them.
- The brothers probably make snide remarks at the love-shy brother's lack of assertiveness and imply that he isn't one of them, say he will die a virgin, and perhaps suggest that he is gay.
- They are usually loners in school and do not make friends for fear they will be vulnerable to more teasing and be rejected again.
- They excel in school and may have skipped a grade, so they are in with much older kids.
- They have very high expectations for themselves and their "dream date"—she would be a gorgeous, active socialite who has all the skills they lack, plus legs that go on forever. In reality, they want to ride on her coattail to instant acceptance and popularity, and also to prove to parents and siblings that they are successful.
- If their relationship does break up, a "shy man" may be devastated and severely depressed to the point of being at risk of attempting suicide. The well-meaning family will suggest he take up square dancing or gourmet cooking to meet females and learn to

communicate. They will fix him up with an acceptable potential partner, but he will be unable to carry it off because he lacks the social skills.

Your problem is not something you can cure all by yourself. It is important that you find a good therapist who can help you develop your potential. So start your search now.

And while you are waiting for an appointment, there are a few things you can do for yourself. Keep a journal; any old notebook that you can use to write out thoughts and feelings is fine. Do not worry about good English, grammar, or punctuation. Nobody is going to read this but you. Keeping a journal is very therapeutic because it encourages you to think freely about your feelings and reactions. You will also find that once you have written out your fears and feelings of inadequacy, all of a sudden, a pattern emerges. You gain real insight into the causes and effects of your behavior. Then you are ready when a therapist makes some suggestions.

Family and roommates must understand that a journal is private and they have absolutely no right to read it. If they do, they are responsible for their reactions.

Keep your journals. It is great therapy to read them over later, to see how you are moving and how far you have progressed. And if you regress, you can go back and work your way out of the slump. When your thoughts and feelings keep going around and around in your head, writing them down reduces their power to keep you off balance, and you become less preoccupied with those feelings.

There are some great books you can get. These are not cheap, and they are not available in most bookstores, so you have to special order them, but they are well worth the effort. They include *The Shy Man Syndrome* by Dr. Brian Gilmartin (Lanham, Md.: Madison Books, 1989), and two other good books by David D. Burns, M.D.: *Intimate Connections: The Clinically Proven Program for Making Close Friends and Finding a Loving Partner* (New York: NAL, 1986), and *Ten Days to Self-Esteem* (New York: Quill, 1999).

Nobody said this would be fast and easy. But, hey, it is worth it. This is the rest of your life we are dealing with. So what are you waiting for?

SMOKING

Dear Sue: *I used to love my husband a great deal, but lately his two-pack-a-day habit is just turning me off. Give me some ammunition I can use to get him to stop.*

Sue says: I used to smoke, so I know that all the ammunition, threats, and warnings about the danger to his health and the cost, as well as the complaint that kissing a smoker is like kissing the bottom of an ashtray, do not have much effect. You can only hope they will all be stored in his memory and that something will happen—a lingering cough, an asthma attack, a cancer scare, and then he will decide, enough . . . It has to be his personal decision, when he is ready. I quit smoking every Monday morning for twenty years. Suddenly, finally, that was it, over and done with.

Here are a few little-known facts:

- Males who smoke are much more likely to become impotent because smoking reduces the circulation of the blood to the penis.
- Smoking adversely affects men's sperm; it decreases their motility, changes their shape, and reduces production.

- Smoking is one of the main contraindications for women going on and staying on the birth-control pill because it dramatically increases the risk of a heart attack or stroke. This also applies to hormone replacement therapy for menopausal women.
- Babies born to mothers who smoked during pregnancy are smaller, less active, and already addicted to nicotine.
- Children raised in families in which either or both parents smoke are much more prone to developing respiratory distress, colds, coughs, and asthma than other kids.

There are some other little-known facts about the effect of smoking on women's fertility:

- Women who smoke are three times more likely to be infertile. They produce less estrogen and do not ovulate regularly. It takes much longer for them to conceive and they are more prone to miscarriages. If they do deliver, their babies will be smaller and more vulnerable to asthma and emphysema.
- Smoking partially paralyzes the cilia in the fallopian tubes, so an egg may be fertilized but it will not be pushed forward to the uterus by the cilia. Therefore, an ectopic pregnancy is more likely.

We all know the statistics on lung cancer for both men and women. More women are smoking more, and there has been a dramatic increase in lung cancer among women.

I assume you have nattered and "bitched" about your husband's smoking, and tried reasoning, threatening, and everything short of moving out. His habit is endangering your health and the children's; insist that he smoke outside. And for every cent he spends on cigarettes, put an equal amount into your wardrobe or toward a trip with the kids or something you really want that does not include the smoker.

The nicotine patch, nicotine gum, and a prescribed medication called Zyban, taken daily, reduce and eventually kill your desire to smoke. But these are effective only if he is ready to quit smoking. But you can't push a chain. He will do it when he is ready, on his terms. Then be prepared for one irritable guy for a few months, but it will be worth it.

STERILIZATION

Dear Sue: My wife and I had three boys, and last month we finally got our girl. We both agree—no more, not now, not ever. We were thinking of sterilization, but we were wondering which one was most effective and easiest.

Sue says: Congratulations on all counts. That's a great family, and I am impressed by your willingness to research, discuss, and agree. So here goes.

Female sterilization is called tubal ligation. It is done in a hospital under general anesthetic, usually by a gynecologist, although in small centers where gynecologists are not available, some family physicians could perform this surgery.

The doctor makes two half-inch incisions, one in the navel and one in the appendix area. A laparoscope (a long, thin tube that has a retractable light, scalpel, and forceps) is used to find the fallopian tubes, which are either cut and tied or "zapped" with an electric cautery. The incision is sutured and the woman stays in the hospital overnight. She is likely fine, but she may be uncomfortable for a few days. No sex until after she has had her period again.

A vasectomy, surgical sterilization on a man, is a very simple surgical procedure performed under local anesthetic in the doctor's office. It may be done by a urologist (specialist in the urinary system), but it can also be performed by your family doctor.

The procedure takes only fifteen minutes. The doctor freezes a small area on either side of the scrotum and makes a small incision on each side. After locating the vas (the small tube that connects the testicle to the urethra), the doctor ties this tube in two spots and cuts between the tie and returns the ends inside the scrotum and sutures up the incision.

The patient goes home following the procedure. He may be uncomfortable, so sitting around with an ice pack on his crotch (a bag of frozen peas works well) is the best thing to do. His testicles will develop some bruising, so they will turn delicate shades of purple, orange, yellow, green, black, and blue. The bruising will fade in about ten to fourteen days.

However, after a vasectomy the couple must continue their regular method of birth control for one month. Then the doctor will check the man's ejaculate to ensure that no sperm are present. When an examination shows the male is "shooting blanks," other methods of birth control can be discontinued. Today a vasectomy can be reversed by microsurgery. The success rate is about 50 percent.

In 1993, controversial research indicated that men who have had a vasectomy had an increased risk of cancer of the prostate. That research has since been refuted.

Medically, a vasectomy is much cheaper and easier than a tubal ligation. But some men are convinced that a vasectomy would emasculate them, that they would be unable to have erections. If a man continues to believe this in spite of updated information, a vasectomy is probably not advisable—his fears would become a self-fulfilling prophecy.

Dear Sue: *I had a tubal ligation about three years ago, and now I really want to have another baby. So I have had the reversal surgery and a few months later I still have not become pregnant. What could be wrong?*

Sue says: Well, there could be a lot of possibilities. If you are over thirty years old, you may not ovulate every month, so let's not give up on a baby yet.

The inside of the fallopian tube is only as thick as the lead of a lead pencil. You can imagine how difficult it would be to suture the edges of two ends together without closing off the channel through the middle in reversal surgery. That requires surgical skill and delicate microsurgery.

The other part of the picture is how much of the tube was damaged and how much of it remains. Normally, the tube is about thirteen centimeters long. If the doctor has been able to save five centimeters, the success rate is very good, but anything under three centimeters has an 18 percent success rate.

Check with your doctor so you have some idea of what your chances are, and don't give up.

Dear Sue: *I never used to have cramps, but since I had my tubal ligation I have had cramps like you wouldn't believe—we are talking killer cramps. How come?*

Sue says: This is not uncommon. Between 10 and 20 percent of women who have been sterilized develop severe menstrual cramps. Researchers believe that the surgery may alter the production of prostaglandins, which makes the uterus contract, causing cramps. Your doctor may prescribe antiprostaglandin medication to stop the cramps.

STRETCH MARKS

Dear Sue: *Having three babies has taken its toll on my body. The thing that bothers me the most are the stretch marks on my breasts, my abdomen, and my hind end. Is there anything I can do to get rid of these ugly silver-gray shriveled lines?*

Sue says: Both males and females can get stretch marks, or *striae distenae,* with weight gain or loss or rapid muscle development resulting from exercise, and females can get them during pregnancy. The underlying tissue gets stretched and does not regain its twang when you lose weight. You end up with thin wavy pale lines that mar your smooth marble flesh, primarily on your breasts, abdomen, hips, and thighs.

There is very little you can do to prevent stretch marks. You can buy creams to rub on—aloe vera or vitamin E cream, and now there is a vitamin-A cream, which some people claim will smooth out these lines. This cream used to be available only by prescription, but now the strength has been reduced and it is available over the counter. Like most creams, it is virtually useless. Do not use vitamin A cream if there is any possibility that you might be pregnant.

Could you regard these stretch marks as a badge of honor? You earned them and you deserve them. You have either lost a great deal of weight, or you have a beautiful new baby, or you got your body back in shape, and this is your medal.

Granted, you never see Miss July, the centerfold of *Play-boy*, with great stretch marks. She probably has them painted over by airbrush so that they are not visible.

SYPHILIS

Dear Sue: *My partner has a mysterious open wet sore on his testicles. Should I be worried?*

Sue says: We thought syphilis had been eradicated, but it has reappeared as yet another STIs. Syphilis is spread by skin to skin contact, generally sexual, although it may be transmitted by oral contact if one of the participants has a chancre. The chancre may be found on or in the vagina and genitals, or the rectum, nipples, or mouth.

A chancre is a dime-sized, painless, raised sore. The center is shallow and will have a serous fluid that is loaded with the bacteria. The first signs will be the appearance of a chancre, then a low-grade fever, general malaise, and perhaps a rash. This clears up but the bacteria are in the body where it may attack the nerves, vision, hearing, brain, or heart. This is called the latent period and the disease will not be diagnosed unless a blood test is done.

After about twenty years, signs and symptoms of tertiary syphilis may appear. Psychiatric problems called general paresis of the insane (or delusions of grandeur), or a "flap foot gait" called tabes dorsalis. It may also cause blindness or a heart condition.

Upon confirmation of a pregnancy, women must have a blood test for syphilis. We can treat syphilis immediately upon diagnosis, but we cannot repair the damage that has already been done. If a pregnant woman has untreated syphilis, the baby may be born blind, covered with a wet rash, or stillborn.

Treatment is free and comes in the form of massive doses of antibiotics over a period of time. The best way to prevent syphilis is to know your partner's past sexual history and ensure that both you and your partner have bloods test taken. A condom provides limited protection.

[t]

THREESOMES

A threesome, or ménage a trois, sounds like great fun and is a fairly common fantasy for many men. Some women really get off on having another partner participate in making love. Others are not convinced that this would be as wonderful as their partner suggests, but get involved and accept or enjoy it. Other women simply reject the idea outright.

Dear Sue: My boyfriend and I have been together for four years, and lately he has been suggesting that we include another person when we have sex. I want to please him but I am not sure how I feel about it. Is it safe?

Sue says: The fact that your partner trusted you enough to share his fantasy with you says a lot about your relationship. And although he is checking it out, he is not pressuring you, which makes it easier. Also, the fact that you did not react negatively and reject the idea outright tells us that you are not locked into a rigid value system. So before we go into the feeling component, let's think about some questions.

Who chooses that other person, you or your partner? Would this person be one of your friends or will you locate someone from a Companions Wanted ad? Are you going to interview the person ahead of time? Are you assertive enough to really check out the possibility of STDs? What about AIDS? Has this person ever done drugs with a needle? Is there a possibility that they have been involved in high-risk sexual behavior without protection? You both must insist on practicing Safer Sex, using condoms. Will you and your partner discuss and agree on exactly what types of sex you will be involved in, whether oral, vaginal, and/or anal intercourse? Will your partner respect your request to stop anytime? Have you agreed if this other person will be a male or a female?

It is nice that you want to please your partner, but how do *you* really feel about this arrangement? Might you feel inadequate if she is gorgeous or is a wild woman in bed? Would you fear that your partner would fall for her and exclude you?

If this other person is a woman, how will you feel about your lover having sex with another woman with you present? And how will you feel if she is kissing and touching you sexually while he is kissing and touching her?

If the other is a male, how will you feel having sex with another guy while your partner looks on, cheering you on? Might you be concerned that your partner has latent homosexual tendencies if he is involved with another guy?

Is there a niggling fear in the back of your mind that your partner might get hooked on this and want to do it all the time? Or the fear that this is just the beginning and might escalate to foursomes, swinging, orgies, bondage, or S&M, just to satisfy his fantasies?

Will you respect him afterward, and will he respect you? Is there a possibility that you might be haunted by flashbacks in the future?

I always find it interesting that males who want to initiate threesomes usually want another female, not another guy. Would the prospect of having another guy actively participating make your boyfriend feel inept and inadequate and give rise to fears of failure? If it would be all right for him to want another female, why would it not be all right if you want another male?

If your relationship breaks up after having had a threesome, how will you feel? And if you agree to this idea just to keep the relationship going because he is implying that you are a prig, you don't need me to tell you that it will break up anyhow, leaving your self-concept and self-esteem badly battered. This is a decision that you have to make thoughtfully and carefully, not just to please him, but based on what is best for you.

TIPPED UTERUS

Dear Sue: *My doctor says I have a tipped uterus. I am eighteen years old. Will it ever straighten up?*

Sue says: A retroverted, or tipped, uterus is one that tilts back toward your spine. It is not uncommon. One in seven women has a retroverted uterus; some are positioned straight up and down, and some tilt forward. Many teenage females have a retroverted uterus. When some girls go through puberty, their uterus grows so fast that the muscles are unable to keep it up. As they mature, the muscles strengthen, and they are fine.

A retroverted uterus may affect your sexual pleasure, and it may make becoming pregnant more difficult. If sex is uncomfortable, try the doggie position, and if you are having difficulty getting pregnant, have sex in the doggie position. You will likely be able to carry a pregnancy to term and deliver a normal, healthy baby.

So please do not get upset or worried, but do see your doctor, who may refer you to a gynecologist. If necessary, surgery is available to hoist your uterus to a normal position.

TOUCHING

We talk about the healing touch, but we forget to use it unless we are reminded, "I need a hug." I have heard it said that we all need four hugs a day to survive, eight to thrive, and twelve to blossom and flourish. But nonsexual human contact is often misinterpreted.

Dear Sue: My husband's family never showed affection for one another, so he will not touch me or the kids except in rough-house play. My family were always touching and hugging, and I hug our kids and give them a backrub at bedtime, but I miss holding my husband. We hugged when we were courting, but now the only time he hugs or kisses me is when he wants sex.

Sue says: Your husband, like so many other men, places the wrong meaning on skin-to-skin contact. We know that little baby boys do not get the same amount of hugging and nuzzling, rocking and cooing, as little girls. At story time, little girls sit on our lap, little boys beside us. Grandma kisses granddaughter, but Grandpa shakes his grandson's hand like a real little man. By age ten, girls still hug and kiss parents, hold hands with their best friends; boys roll their eyes back in their head and avoid all contact with anybody, fearful it would be interpreted as "mama's-boy" or "fag" behavior.

During adolescence, males start having serious spontaneous erections. This embarrasses them because it can happen for no reason at all but is guaranteed to happen if they touch a girl. So touch becomes equated with sex. When a teenage boy is dating, holding hands is regarded as an overture to sex, and if she hugs and kisses him, he translates that into consenting to go further, all the way, if he can.

Unless she stops him, that pattern continues in the relationship, so if she hugs him close, he thinks, "She must want it." If he continues to make sexual moves and she agrees, it worked. If she does not respond, he feels rejected and is reluctant to try again.

This is why I get letters such as this one:

Dear Sue: *My husband never wants to just hug and cuddle and kiss. He always interprets it as an invitation to sex. Meanwhile, I just want to snuggle. As a result, I avoid all body contact with him, but I miss it.*

Sue says: Most couples develop other cues and clues that indicate they would like to "fool around." It may be a wink, a knowing look, a pelvic, grinding hug, or a French kiss; they both know what the message is and may consent or say, "Not tonight, dear." For them, hugs and snuggles happen all the time, doing the dishes, watching TV—anytime is a good time. Their kids see this, are used to it, and it will become routine for them. For other couples, a hug is interpreted as an invitation to initiate sex.

Communication skills come into play here. If you can use "I" terms, saying, "Remember when we were going out together and we used to hug all the time. I really liked it, and now I miss that contact. Could we find a different signal to initiate sex, and keep on hugging and kissing as often as possible?"

I am willing to bet he would be delighted, because, basically, males need and like body contact every bit as much as females do. If you have difficulty convincing him, you may need a few sessions with a good counselor who can help the two of you develop essential communication skills. Then you can give him a back rub and he won't be expecting sex. Watch him purr.

TRUST

If a relationship is to last, there must be a high degree of trust. This involves more than knowing that your partner will not be "messing around" on you. You also need to know that neither of you will betray the intimate aspects of yourselves or your relationship to anyone else.

Dear Sue: My girlfriend and I have been living together for four years now. It's been good, but lately she has been talking "baby." She is thirty-five and says her biological clock is ticking, and she is into nesting. Not me—that's the last thing I need right now. She is on the Pill, and I am scared that she will "accidentally" forget a few pills, get pregnant, and insist on having the baby. She got real upset when I suggested we use condoms, so right now I am reluctant to have sex with her. She is wondering if I still love her. I'm feeling like I have no say in the matter and I'm terrified I'll be trapped.

Sue says: This is crazy-making for you. You do not have a choice—you must sit down and be very open. Using "I" terms (putting the emphasis on how you feel, not what she's doing), tell her very clearly exactly how you feel and what your bottom line is. This sounds ruthless, but she needs to know. You can tell her that you do *not* want to be a father, and you are not sure you ever will want to have a family. She must be aware that if having a baby is her number one priority, it would be best to end the relationship right now.

But what if she decided to get pregnant in spite of your refusal? You would be powerless. All she has to do is go off the Pill, and you would never know. You are, indeed, powerless. She could pressure you (con you?) into sex, get pregnant (by you or by somebody else—that has happened before). Legally, you could not force her to terminate the pregnancy. If she had the baby, the relationship would probably break up. But she could charge you for child support until the child was an adult. Are we surprised when you say you do not want to have sex?

If you have analyzed it honestly, you know the relationship is already in deep trouble. The trust level is almost nonexistent and you are starting to be evasive. Being very honest with your feelings may jeopardize your relationship even more, but if you want guarantees, you are going to have to insist on using condoms, although even that is not without some risk.

The harsh reality is, even if you stopped having sex completely, it would be your word against hers. Legally, you could go to court, get a court order for a DNA blood test to establish paternity. By this time the relationship would have gone down the tubes.

The whole prospect is enough to scare many men off if they do not want to be a father in the near future. I'm convinced this is a deep fear that many males have—no power, no control over the final outcome of an unplanned pregnancy. This fact may explain why males are reluctant to commit to a relationship, why they suffer many of the common sexual dysfunctions such as delayed ejaculation, impotence, or premature ejaculation.

"Fear" is the operative word. The absence of trust guarantees fear. Another stumbling block—once trust has been damaged, can you ever really get it back? I have a feeling that you have a gut sense of what would be best for you, and writing it out in a journal may help to clarify it.

Dear Sue: *I made a big mistake. Although my boyfriend says he forgives me, I know he hasn't forgotten. Our friends say he is always checking up on me.*

Sue says: It is almost impossible for a person who has been deceived or hurt to just forget it. But we do have control over our reaction and response to an unpleasant memory. Your boyfriend can acknowledge the mistake, accept that you are sincerely sorry and that it will not happen again, ever, and consciously decide to move past this error in judgment and start to build trust again. You have to prove you are worthy of that trust.

But if your partner uses that as a weapon, constantly reminding you of your boo boo, holding it over your head, or using it to make you feel inadequate, that error becomes a major club for control and power.

Reminding this partner that he is not perfect and that he has pulled a few "rank" ones in his day will not succeed. This will just leave you feeling guilty and angry. It would be natural for you to criticize him to try to get even. Then we would be into playing games and scoring points.

It is difficult to communicate your feelings because this partner might build on your feelings of failure. I suggest you go for relationship counseling. Your partner is holding on to power and needs to deal with that, or it will come out in other ways in the relationship.

I do not want you feeling you have to pay for the rest of your life for an error in judgment that you have acknowledged.

I firmly believe in working things through, but only if it pays off, the issue gets resolved, put behind you, and you move on together.

Used as a weapon, this feeling of never quite being forgiven may be very damaging to your self-concept and self-esteem. It can leave you vulnerable to mental, physical, or sexual abuse by your partner because you are convinced that you do not deserve any better. So you made a mistake; it is not terminal, and you deserve to be able to learn from it and not have your nose rubbed in it all the time. Do go for counseling.

[u]

UNCONSUMMATED SEX

Dear Sue: *My wife and I are from the same religious back-ground and culture. When we were dating, I respected her, and we did not "do" anything. On our honeymoon, she was nervous and scared and exhausted. I was hungover from my stag the night before, so I didn't try anything. After that we would hug and kiss and a bit of petting, but the minute I got aroused, she would push me away. We have now been married for eighteen months and have never had sexual inter-course. Neither of us had any sex education at home or at school. It was assumed that when the time came I would know exactly what to do, and she thought her husband would teach her all she ever needed to know about sex. I know it is as much my fault as hers, but I do not want this to continue. I have never told anybody about this before. I am so embarrassed.*

Sue says: I really appreciate how much courage it took to write this letter. I am sending it back to you, and I want you to give it to your wife to read. I hope this will open it up for discussion. Tell her how you are feeling, besides embarrassed. Perhaps you are also feeling inadequate as a man and as a husband; you may feel frustrated, angry at yourself and at her, ashamed, foolish, fearful that you will never get it together; and you may feel trapped because you both made vows, "for better for worse, till death do us part." When you tell her how you are feeling, you are not blaming her, but simply saying that this is how you are affected. Then ask her how she feels about it.

I want you to go to a bookstore where you will not be recognized and get *The New Male Sexuality* by Bernie Zilbergeld, Ph.D. (New York: Bantam, 1999), and *The Magic of Sex* by Miriam Stoppard (New York: Penguin, 2001). Read these books yourself, then read them aloud together and share your thoughts. This will be a whole new learning experience for both of you.

It might not be a bad idea if your wife went to her family doctor for a pelvic examination to be certain everything is normal and to choose a good method of birth control.

Go slow and easy. You have waited eighteen months, and she will not become "the last of the red hot mamas" overnight, and that's good because you will not be a Don Juan either. Not yet . . .

If it is just not happening, find a good sex therapist and get individual and conjoint sex counseling. Don't make this a chore. Enjoy. Getting there is half the fun.

For the following couple, getting there was no fun:

Dear Sue: *My girlfriend was the victim of childhood incest. So we can kiss and neck and do a bit of petting, but if I go any* *further, she gets all upset and cries and locks herself in the bathroom. I love her and want to marry her, but I cannot compete with the ghost of her stepbrother in our bedroom. She says she is getting over it and by the time we get married, she will be okay.*

Sue says: Please, read the section on sexual assault on page 245 to become aware of what is happening to her as a result of her early sexual experiences. You will also learn that she must get counseling if she is to move from the victim to the survivor stage. Knowing that, you can be a supportive and empathic listener. You cannot rescue her, but you can be there for her.

This experience has probably made you very aware of the trauma caused by all forms of sexual assault, so you will not tolerate sexist remarks and jokes in the future.

Dear Sue: *I am simply unable to have sex with my wife. It is not because she is unwilling, but she has two very small vaginal openings, two vaginas parallel to each other, beginning halfway up by the cervix. She never could get a tampon in, but she figured that was because she was a virgin. I discovered the two openings when we were petting and I realized I had one finger in each opening. Sure surprised me. Now what?*

Sue says: She will have to go to her family doctor for a pelvic exam. The doctor will confirm your diagnosis of a bifurcated vagina and refer her to a gynecologist. Under general anesthetic, they will open up the hymen, remove the membrane dividing the vaginal canal, make sure there is no bleeding, and she will be fine.

The doctor will give her instructions to use her fingers, well lubricated, three times a day to stretch the vagina to prevent it from healing together again. Not painful, but essential.

The doctor will tell you when you can have sex; then use a condom to prevent infection, and do be gentle.

She will probably be able to deliver a baby through the vagina, and she will be fine.

UTERINE ABLATION

Dear Sue: I have had heavy, heavy bleeding from my vagina for about two months. I was referred to a gynecologist, who did a routine D&C. But the bleeding continued, so now they are talking about doing a uterine ablation. What is this?

Sue says: A D&C cleans out the endometrial lining of the uterus, which generally stops the bleeding. However, if it continues, in the past the doctor would have performed a hysterectomy. Now the doctor may examine the inside of your uterus with a hysteroscope, and then using either a laser beam or cautery, he will burn off the old lining down to healthy tissue. You will have bleeding and discharge for a few weeks. After that, things will probably settle down and you will be fine. (Eighty percent of women who have this procedure notice significant improvement in their bleeding.)

Because this procedure causes extensive scarring, you will not be able to have more children, but it may allow you to avoid a hysterectomy.

[v]

VAGINAL FARTS

Dear Sue: *Sometimes when my boyfriend and I have sex, I make awful sounds like farting, and I am so embarrassed that I make him stop. Am I losing control?*

Sue says: Honey, you never had control over vaginal farts. When you and your boyfriend are having intercourse, his penis thrusting into your vagina acts like a piston, forcing air up into your vagina. This is a dead-end street and it is not going anywhere, so when the pressure builds up, it has to escape.

There is no sphincter (a tight round band of muscles) to clamp down the vaginal opening. This air is not quiet when it "fluffs" out—it blasts. One lady told me that she blew her partner's penis right out of her vagina. There is nothing you can do but laugh at yourself, and you will find that the more you laugh, the more you fart. So just let go and enjoy. (Vaginal farts don't smell like the other kind.)

VIRGINITY

Dear Sue: *Am I still a virgin? I have never had sex, but I have done everything else.*

Sue says: Absolutely. This applies to both males and females. A virgin is a person who has never had sexual intercourse. So, technically, you are still a virgin. Many teens have anal sex, claiming they want to remain a virgin, and also to avoid pregnancy. Problem: if any of his ejaculate comes in contact with the mucous membrane of her vagina, the sperm can swim and she can get pregnant. Another virgin birth.

Dear Sue: *Is there any way you can regain your virginity?*

Sue says: No, once you have had sexual intercourse, you are no longer a virgin. Now, I have heard of women going to unscrupulous doctors to have their hymen stitched tighter again so she, for religious or cultural reasons, could claim she was a virgin when she got married.

There are a few fundamentalist churches that have a "revirginization" ceremony, which cleanses and purifies you if you regret that you had sex. But technically, you are still not a virgin.

The *Janus Report on Sexual Behavior* by Samuel S. Janus, Ph.D., and Cynthia L. Janus, M.D. (New York: Wiley, 1994) is comparable to the *Kinsey Report* of the late 1940s. This report says that most females regarded virginity after age eighteen as a liability, and something they were in a hurry to lose. This is a dramatic shift in attitude about the importance of virginity until marriage.

Dear Sue: *Can you tell if a guy is a virgin? My boyfriend insists he is, but I do not believe him.*

Sue says: It is impossible to tell for sure if a male is still a virgin, although you may suspect it is true if he appears to be totally inexperienced, but males can be great actors, too. My concern is, is he trying to convince you he has never had sex, and therefore he could not possibly have any diseases, including AIDS, and therefore does not have to practice Safer Sex? You never know, so do not take chances. You can tell him that you are no virgin, so you insist on protecting him. No excuses, practice Safer Sex. Condoms.

Dear Sue: *I have had sex before but my girlfriend hasn't, and no matter how relaxed she is and how much lubrication we use, I simply cannot penetrate her. What's wrong?*

Sue says: Nothing is wrong, but her hymen may be very dense tissue that resists stretching and has not split. Please do not continue to attempt intercourse because it will be painful, and then she will tense up, resulting in more pain, and eventually she will start avoiding sex altogether. This is called dyspareunia.

She should explain the problem to her family doctor, who will do a pelvic examination to see if the hymen is resistant. If so, the doctor will use a local anesthetic and make a very small incision into the hymen, thus widening the opening. It will take about two weeks to heal, so no sexual contact during that time because of the risk of infection. Then do use condoms and lots of lubrication, and be sure she is relaxed and she wants to have sex. This is important because if she still anticipates pain, she will tense up and tighten her pubococcygeus muscles, so sex will not be great. She can gradually learn to relax and comfortably enjoy a penis in her vagina. If not, she might need to see a good gynecologist, who may refer her to a sex therapist.

Dear Sue: *Every time we have sex, there is a lot of bright blood around my girlfriend's vagina. Why?*

Sue says: I'm not sure, but it could be one of several things. Perhaps she has a blood vessel right at the surface of her vaginal opening. It may be getting stretched or the friction may cause it to break open again and bleed. She should go to her doctor, who will probably cauterize it, close it off, and she will be fine.

Another possibility may be that your foreskin is tight and it tears a little bit and bleeds every time you have sex.

Bright bleeding is fresh blood, not old menstrual blood left over, so we know it is near the opening. But if this has been a long-standing problem, it is a nuisance and it can be scary, so why not have it checked out?

[y]

YEAST INFECTION

Dear Sue: *I had a lot of thick white gloopy discharge from my vagina, so I went to the doctor and he diagnosed a "yeast infection." Yech. My boyfriend and I are each other's first lover, so I know it is not an STI, but I feel so dirty and guilty. Where did this infection come from?*

Sue says: Vaginal yeast infections are so common personally, I do not know one woman who has not had an infection at least once. You see, the yeast spores are normally found in the vagina, but every once in a while they overgrow or go crazy. We are not 100 percent sure what triggers this; some say stress, some say diet; definitely the birth-control pill, antibiotics, and frequent sexual activity after a period of abstinence all contribute to the condition.

The first symptom is a thick, white, clumpy, creamy discharge. The vagina burns and itches, gets raw, red, and so irritated that you walk funny. You just want to sit in a nice tub of cool water, and you certainly do not want sex!

Please do not feel guilty or ashamed. This is so common, doctors are quite blasé about it. If there are any other women out there with these symptoms, you should phone your doctor, describe the symptoms, and ask for a quickie appointment because you are miserable. Do not take a bath just before you go to the doctor because you will wash away all the discharge, making it difficult to do a test and make a diagnosis. The doctor will probably prescribe either three or seven white vaginal suppositories that look like white plastic bullets. Expensive at around twenty-five dollars, but you need them.

That night, before you go to bed, have a bath, and then insert one of these suppositories up as far as it will go into your vagina. Wear a minipad because you may drip. While you sleep, the suppository will dissolve, the medication will kill off the spores, and by morning, after a shower, you will feel normal. Do wear a minipad during the day.

Just because you feel better does not mean the infection is under control. You must use all the suppositories as prescribed. Otherwise the yeast will flare up all over again.

Although the flare-up is under control, your vagina is still very raw, sore and irritated, and vulnerable to repeat infection, so doctors recommend that you abstain from intercourse for about a week to ten days. Your partner must use condoms for at least a week after that. Sounds like punishment, but actually the yeast spores can hide under his foreskin, and if you have unprotected sex, they can set off another round of infection.

An oral antifungal medication called Diflucan may be prescribed for chronic yeast infections. See your doctor.

Dear Sue: *Can guys get yeast infections, too?*

Sue says: Not as such, but guys can harbor the spores under their foreskin, so they must retract the foreskin and wash with soap and water when showering. If your partner has a yeast infection and you have sex, the mucous membrane of the head of your penis may become dry, cracked, red, irritated, and sore.

If this happens, make an appointment with your doctor, who will probably prescribe an antifungal cream to rub on twice a day. Apply some cream under the foreskin, too. As a precaution, do use a condom till you are both back to roaring normal again.

Dear Sue: *I have an ongoing yeast infection. I get it treated to the tune of twenty-five dollars; then in a week it is back again. Is there anything I can do to get rid of it forever?*

Sue says: Well, maybe not forever, but there are a few things you can do so you don't get it as frequently. Next flare-up, go to your drugstore for seven-day antifungal suppositories, which is renewable once. That will give you seven suppositories rather than the three. Use one a day, as directed for seven nights.

You still have the other seven suppositories. Use one after sex just to keep the yeast from flaring up again. And because many women have an outbreak during or immediately after their menstrual period, use one suppository at the onset of your period and one the night it is finished. Sounds like a nuisance, and it is, but if it helps, it will be worth it.

At the same time, change a few things in your life:

- Every day eat one or two 250-gram tub(s) of all-natural yogurt that contains no sugar, no fruit, and no starch or gelatin thickener. You'll get to like it—

honestly. You may have to search for it—not all health-food stores sell it.

- Have a bath instead of a shower every day—much more soothing for your genitals. No soap because that is irritating.
- Do not wear panties with a nylon or Lycra crotch unless there is a cotton liner. Try to stay away from panty hose because they are snug and keep body heat around your crotch, which promotes yeast overgrowth.
- Cut down on the amount of sugars and starches in your diet (bread, sweet desserts).
- Some women keep yeast infections under control by taking (orally) an acidophilus capsule every day.
- Others insert a capsule into their vagina at night to dissolve and change the acid/alkaline balance of the vagina and clear the infection.
- Some women spoon one tablespoon or more of plain, unsweetened natural yogurt into their vagina at bedtime, wear a minipad, and have a bath in the morning.
- Please be aware that your sex partner may carry the yeast spores around the head of his penis. Protect yourself—use condoms. He must use an antifungal cream to get rid of the yeast.
- If after all this the yeast infection still returns, you may have to consider going off the birth-control pill. Normally, the vagina has an acid base, which keeps the yeast spores under control. But when you go on the Pill, the vagina changes to alkaline, like soda bicarbonate, instead of vinegar, so the yeast grows out of control. Taking a six-month break from the Pill might be the answer. But before you do this, please

be sure you and your partner replace the Pill with another effective method of contraception.

- If the yeast infection does not respond to vaginal, or local, treatment, ask your doctor for a prescription for Diflucan, an oral antifungal medication.
- Do use condoms until things are under control. I do not want to raise suspicions, but I have heard too many women tell me afterward that their partner was having sex with another person who had yeast and he dutifully brought it home. So, protect yourself.

A word about douching. Most medical professionals will tell you that routine douching for cleanliness is not necessary. In fact, it can be harmful because it changes the acid alkaline balance of your vagina, leaving you vulnerable to infections. Also, douching removes the normal bacteria present in the vagina.

But many doctors suggest buying a douche nozzle at your drugstore. Pour one-quarter cup of vinegar in with two cups of warm water and use that as a douche before you go to bed if you suspect you might be getting an infection. Do not use the commercial douche preparations. They are expensive and no more effective than your own do-it-yourself preparation. If you have bought one, save the nozzle and plastic bottle to reuse with vinegar and water. Recycle, yes, but be sure to wash this equipment well to prevent reinfection.

Now, I really do not want to scare you, but we are becoming more aware that if a female has HIV, which causes AIDS, she has altogether different symptoms than males do. Women have severe chronic ongoing gynecological problems, prolonged painful periods, endometriosis, ovarian cysts, and yeast infections from hell. So if you have severe yeast that does not respond to treatment, and if you are at risk (that means if you have done heavy-duty injectable drugs, had unprotected sex with a high-risk partner, or had a blood transfusion during the years 1980 to 1985), ask for an AIDS test. Don't be timid about asking; insist on it. Early treatment of AIDS is important.